FLORIDA

CAREGIVERS HANDBOOK
REVISED SECOND EDITION

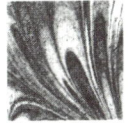

Edited by Creston Nelson-Morrill

An Essential Resource

Guide for Caregivers

& Their Older Loved Ones

Including a Directory of
Services and Support Organizations for the Caregiver

The Florida Caregivers Handbook
An Essential Resource Guide for Caregivers and Their Older Loved Ones
Edited by Creston Nelson-Morrill

Published by HealthTrac Books, Tallahassee

Copyright © 1993 by HealthTrac Research Group, Inc.

All rights reserved under International and Pan-American Copyright Conventions.
No part of this book may be reproduced or transmitted by any means, mechanical
or electronic, without written permission from the author, except for
material to be used in reviews.

ISBN 0-9638162-0-9

Manufactured in the United States of America
Second Edition: September, 1993

10 9 8 7 6 5 4 3 2 1

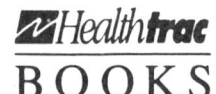
BOOKS
Post Office Box 13599
Tallahassee, FL 32317

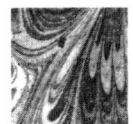

Contents

Foreword v

Acknowledgements vii

Introduction 1

1. Caregiving: The Emotional Rewards and Challenges 7
   Judith A.S. Altholz, Ph.D.

2. Legal Aspects of Caregiving 23
   Tann Hunt, J.D.

3. Ethical Aspects of Caregiving 37
   Margaret Lynn Duggar, M.S., Ed.

4. Long-Distance Caregiving 47
   Marian Bruin, A.C.S.W., B.C.D.

5. Successful Communication 61
   Dawn Pollock and Judith Altholz, Ph.D.

6. Medication Management and the Normal Aging Process 71
   Robert J. Kassan, M.D.

7. Alcohol and Substance Abuse in The Elderly 81
   Jayne LaRue, M.S.W.

8. Dementia and the Caregiver 95
   George F. Slade, M.D.

9. Caring and Grieving 109
   Karen Ring, M.S.W., L.C.S.W.

10. Financial Planning 139
    C. Colburn Hardy

11. The Nursing Home Decision 157
    Pamela Cody

12. Medicare, Medicaid, and Medicare Supplement Insurance 169
    Thomas Walter Poulton

13. The Corporate Response to Caregiving 197
    Marie E. Cowart, R.N., Ph.D.

14. Advocating for the Care Recipient 207
    Creston Nelson-Morrill

15. Navigating the System 225
    Creston Nelson-Morrill

16. Directory of Elder Services
    and Caregiver Support Organizations 235

    About the Contributors 273

    About HealthTrac Research Group 276

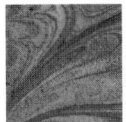

Foreword

It is my privilege to introduce this newest edition of the *Florida Caregivers Handbook*. I believe that caregivers and their families will find this document to be a valuable source of both information and moral support.

As the chairman and chief executive officer of the state's largest electric utility, I am keenly aware of the special needs of many older Floridians. Approximately one of every five persons in our service area is age 65 or older.

One of an electric utility's basic operating principles is the "obligation to serve." Simply stated, we're obliged to provide safe, reliable and affordable electricity to everyone within our service area. But since electricity has become such a necessity in everyday life, this obligation has taken on a broader meaning for us—especially with regard to Florida's older citizens.

Our company works closely with federal, state and local aging organizations in implementing dozens of programs that focus on meeting the fiscal and physical needs of senior citizens. For example, our financial support services include a special payment plan that extends the "payment due" date for those depending on Social Security or similar benefits. And FPL's Quality Senior Living Van brings displays and information on aging right to the older citizen's doorstep.

As with any large company, many of FPL's employees have obligations to care for older family members. Knowing the great physical, financial and emotional toll this can have on our workers, we've offered assistance by helping to set up a special "dependent care account." This program allows employees to set aside money in a tax-free account to use for specified purposes, such as paying for nursing care. FPL also sponsors special "caregiver fairs," which showcase the support services available to FPL employees and retirees in their communities.

FPL is certainly not unique among electric utilities—and other companies—in providing these services. As Florida's older citizens grow in number, however, enhancing their quality of life will become even more important.

At FPL, we pledge our continued support toward caregivers' efforts... and we hope other companies will do the same.

James L. Broadhead

James L. Broadhead
Chairman and CEO
Florida Power & Light Company

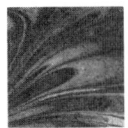

Acknowledgements

We wish to thank the following persons for their help in making the second edition of the *Florida Caregivers Handbook* a reality:

The contributors, who so generously shared their knowledge of elder care and related fields.

FPL Chairman and CEO James Broadhead, for his continuing commitment to older Floridians and their caregivers.

Blue Cross and Blue Shield of Florida President and CEO Bill Flaherty and Florida Hospital Association President Charles S. Pierce, Jr., for their generous support of this project.

And our 1992–93 board chairperson, Doris Reeves-Lipscomb, who has served as the guiding hand as the HealthTrac Research Group has charted its course for the remainder of the decade.

Board of Directors
HealthTrac Research Group

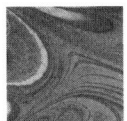

Introduction

Nationally, there are more than 30 million people over the age of 60. In Florida, 23 percent of the population—just over 3 million people—is aged 60 or older. By the year 2000, Florida's older population will reach 3.8 million.

Most older Americans continue to lead active lives. They are healthy and involved in the community. But state revenue estimators predict that by 1995, nearly 270,000 Floridians will be over the age of 85. Twenty-three percent will have four or more limitations on activities of daily living (ADL), which include eating, dressing and personal hygiene. Many will need a caregiver.

A caregiver is someone who provides care to an older, chronically ill, or disabled person in the caregiver's or the care recipient's home or in a long-term care setting. The caregiver of an older person may be the care recipient's spouse, sibling, or child or a close friend or other relative. In rare instances, the caregiver may be the care recipient's parent.

Eighty to ninety percent of the care received by older persons is provided by family and friends. The emotional and physical toll on the principal caregiver is enormous.

Caregiving can include personal care, housekeeping, meal preparation, medication and financial management, running errands and providing transportation. It can involve an hour or less a day, or it can be an all-consuming 24-hour-a-day job. There are few challenges in life more difficult.

The financial status of many older persons complicates matters. In Florida, which leads the nation in its number of older residents as a percentage of total population, more than 327,000 live at or near the poverty level. Sadly, individuals who live below the poverty level are six times more likely to be institutionalized than their more financially able counterparts. In 1993, the poverty level for individuals was an annual income of less than $6,972. The poverty level for couples was $9,432. The Florida Pepper Commission on Aging found that in Florida about one in five women aged 85 or older live in poverty.

In Florida, nearly 70,000 persons are receiving care through community-based care programs; a similar number live in residential room, board, and personal care facilities. Almost 68,000 older Floridians live in nursing homes, with nearly half of them over the age of 85, and at their most vulnerable. Estimates of the number of persons over age 85 who suffer from Alzheimer's disease or related dementia range from one in four to nearly half.

E. Bentley Lipscomb, secretary of the Florida Department of Elder Affairs (DOEA), calls Alzheimer's disease a "coming epidemic." With more than 288,000 cases reported, Florida has a larger Alzheimer's population than the national total of AIDS victims.

There is no law requiring family members to provide care to loved ones afflicted with the disease, Lipscomb notes. If just 15 percent of Alzheimer's victims' caregivers abandoned their loved ones, the cost to the state of Florida in increased nursing home funding would be $1 billion annually, he says.

A national survey cosponsored in 1988 by the American Association of Retired Persons, (AARP) and The Travelers Companies; Older Americans Program found that 7 million households include a caregiver. More than one-half of those households include a working caregiver. Seventy-five percent of caregivers were females, with most under 50 years of age. The median age of caregivers was 45.

The AARP survey also found the following:

- The average age of care recipients was 77. Thirty-one percent of workers were providing care for their mothers.
- Working caregivers averaged about 10 hours weekly on caregiving. But more than one-quarter of full-time workers spent 21 *or more* hours per week on caregiving.
- Most employed caregivers provided assistance with instrumental activities of daily living (ADL), such as grocery shopping, transportation and housekeeping. More than 60 percent also provided assistance with ADL, most involving personal care.

- Twenty-nine percent of the caregivers surveyed lived with the care recipient; 13 percent lived 20 *or more* minutes away.
- Full-time employees used about 5 percent of their monthly incomes to pay for care-related expenses. They spent an average of $475 per month on in-home nursing care, $167 per month on hospital care, and $113 on other expenses.

If the survey tells us nothing else, it tells us that a large number of caregivers are working one and a half jobs when caregiving and employment are taken into account.

Prior to making the decision to enter into a caregiving relationship, potential caregivers may wish to consider the following list of questions:

What is the nature of your relationship with the care recipient? Have you resolved any major differences that you may have had in the past? How do you and the care recipient approach problem resolution (i.e., confrontation, denial, guilt)?

What are the care recipient's or your own physical or mental disabilities or limitations? How do you feel about the care recipient's disabilities?

What is the first word that comes to mind when you think about dealing with the care recipient on a daily basis?

How many people are you taking on in providing care? How will the care recipient's and your own loved ones respond to your new role? What is the potential for conflict among the interested parties?

How many months or years are you willing to play the role of caregiver? What will you do if the care recipient outlives your desire to provide him or her with care?

Can you afford to take on the responsibilities of caregiving? What kind of financial support can you expect from the care recipient? Are there family members who might interfere in the care recipient's and your own financial affairs?

Will the care recipient have to make changes in his or her life that will mean moving away from familiar friends and surroundings? Is he or she likely to feel lonely or isolated?

How well do you and/or the care recipient cope with stress and change?

What alternative arrangements can be made for the care recipient?

For many would-be caregivers, the temptation is to answer the last question by saying that no alternatives to hands-on caregiving exist. The fact is that while they may be less desirable in some respects, there are other options. Many friends and family members of care recipients choose the role of care manager instead. Care management generally does not include the direct provision of personal care services.

Assuming the role of caregiver is a stressful event with the potential for family breakdown. Margaret Awad, an assistant professor in the Florida State University School of Nursing, has said that when families cannot cope with changes and are overwhelmed by their inability to meet demands placed on them by the dependent elderly, they experience a state of crisis. Whether the family assumes the role willingly or reluctantly, it still carries with it the element of stress and is a potential crisis situation, she said.

Even with the potential for crisis, caregiving can be a tremendously rewarding experience. The nature of the experience is dependent upon the complex mix of family values, the extent and nature of the care recipient's incapacity, and the capacity of the caregiver to constantly adapt to new situations and relationships.

Immediate gratification for the caregiver may or may not be a byproduct of the caregiving relationship. The care recipient may be consumed with a feeling of loss over diminished capacity. He or she may resent his or her reliance on you. While some care recipients are grateful for their caregiver's efforts in their behalf, many caregivers never hear the two words they most long to hear: thank you.

In the following chapters we will attempt to define services available to older persons and their caregivers and to unravel the mysteries surrounding the current web of service delivery. At this writing, it appears that major changes are in store for Florida's aging services network when the Legislature convenes in February 1994. The most likely scenario: elderc are services currently located within the Department of Health and Rehabilitative Services will be relocated to the DOEA.

We also will look at the ethical dimensions of caregiving and discuss: the impact of caregiving on the caregiver and his or her family; long-distance caregiving; grieving; dementia; medication management; changes that may occur in the elderly as part of the normal aging process; alcohol and substance abuse; legal considerations; financial planning; communicating with the sensory-impaired or confused older person; the corporate awakening to the impact of caregiving on working caregivers; and advocating for the care recipient.

The late Florida Congressman Claude Pepper, who served in both the U.S. House and Senate for total of more than 50 years, once said, "The young and the old have everything to gain from one another and only need a chance to discover the bond."

In most cases, there is no stronger bond than that between the caregiver and his or her loved one.

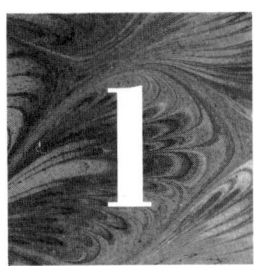

Caregiving: The Emotional Rewards and Challenges

Judith A.S. Altholz, Ph.D.

As a caregiver, your efforts can carry both the great rewards of helping someone you love and the significant challenges of patience and commitment. When we discuss caregiving, we often focus on the person who is receiving care rather than on person who is giving care. While we are concerned about the impact of illness on the recipient, we must remember that the effect of watching a loved one become increasingly disabled can be devastating to the caregiver.

This chapter focuses on the emotional aspects of being a caregiver through an investigation of feelings, beliefs and values associated with:

- the decision to enter into a caregiving relationship;
- the stresses and challenges of daily caregiving; and
- the question of institutionalization.

This chapter is intended to help you better understand the emotional challenges of caregiving and to realize that you are not alone in facing sometimes painful decisions. Caregiving is a complex and demanding task. Hopefully, this chapter will give you a greater understanding and appreciation of yourself.

The Caregiving Decision

The family is most often thought of as providing care for older loved ones. However, the term "caregiver" can be used to describe a variety of persons who may be involved in providing services. An older person may be cared for by a spouse or partner, children, siblings, friends and/or neighbors.

It is true, however, that family members are most likely to provide care for the older person. There is no evidence to support the myth that families tend to "dump" their older members in institutions. In fact, the more common situation is for families to take care of their older family members without assistance until they exhaust themselves emotionally, physically and financially. By the time help is finally sought, the family may no longer be able to provide care at all. A crisis, physical and emotional, is created for both the care recipient and the caregiver.

To be sure, caregiving can be very satisfying. Providing assistance for someone you love and who may have at one time cared for you can sustain and even strengthen the bond with a loved one. The commitments that are made between spouses and partners, or children and parents, are often fulfilled through caregiving. It is important to realize, however, that caregiving can also be a burden that weighs heavily on the caregiver and the family. Whether or not to enter into a caregiving relationship, given the degree of caregiving required, is a decision that raises a number of issues that deserve careful consideration.

THE CAREGIVING RELATIONSHIP

Caregivers often have a variety of feelings about both the person to whom they are providing care and about caregiving itself. Facing the decline of a loved one can be difficult to understand and to accept. Parents, spouses, and friends who were once vigorous and healthy may now be confused and unable to handle the most simple physical and mental tasks. The disabilities of a loved one cause sadness as we remember the way the person used to be and recognize the hopelessness of recovery. The caregiver may fear further decline and additional responsibility, wondering if it is possible to do more than he or she is already doing.

Illness and disability can rekindle or evoke feelings of anger and resentment. Frequently, caregivers have additional caregiving responsibilities to a spouse or to children. The question "When will I get time for me?" is not easily answered in the face of possible 24-hour responsibility. All of these feelings are natural and need to be considered during the caregiving decision-making process. Sometimes people do not express these "negative" concerns because they believe that they should not feel this way. But feelings are neither "right" nor "wrong," "good" nor "bad"—they simply are. They provide us with information about ourselves.

It is extremely important to allow ourselves to become aware of how we feel and to ask ourselves what these emotions mean. Realistic appraisal of your ability to be a caregiver is critical. It is not fair to yourself or to the care recipient to enter into a caregiving relationship because you feel you "should" if you do not think you "can." It is far better to make arrangements with other family members or community agencies to make sure that needed care is provided, rather than to take on a role that may be destructive both to you and to the recipient.

THE CAREGIVING ENVIRONMENT

The Care Recipient's Home

As a caregiver, you may find yourself in the position of caring for an older person who still lives in his or her own home. You may have concerns about safety and crime, forgetfulness, nutrition, medication, exercise and physical health. You may wonder if the recipient should continue to live alone or if it is time for a change in living arrangements.

It is important to view the older person and the issue of care and the environment as realistically as possible. Issues that are of concern to you may not be of concern to the care recipient. He or she may believe that the benefits of staying at home outweigh the drawbacks.

For example, let us assume that your widowed father is living in the same house that he and your mother bought 50 years before. Over time, the neighborhood has deteriorated and is no longer as safe as it once was. Many of your father's friends have died or moved away, although a few still live close by. You find yourself worrying constantly about whether your father will be mugged when he goes outside. You might wonder what would happen if he fell, how long it would take for him to be found, and who would find him.

Your father, on the other hand, still feels comfortable in the neighborhood and does not want to leave the house in which he and your mother were so happy. He still has a few close friends whom he visits daily. He says that they would know that something was wrong if he one day failed to visit. Perhaps the neighborhood is not as safe as it once was, he concedes, but he is at home there and would feel lost and alone if he were to leave.

Although you would feel much better having your father in a safer neighborhood, perhaps closer to you, it is critical to balance his needs and wants with your concerns. This would be a perfect time to sit down together and realistically discuss the future. What would happen if he did fall and break a hip? How long might it be before he was found? Perhaps it would put your mind—and his—at ease if he would agree to use a telephone reassurance service, a community-based program that would call him each day at the same time to make sure that he is safe and well.

If he should have to leave his home, where would your father want to go? We are often very reluctant to discuss openly a future that may include increasing frailty, illness, and need for care. It is almost as if we believe that if we refuse to talk about these realities, they will not occur. Unfortunately, these issues frequently are not raised until a crisis arises that demands immediate action. Long-term care decisions are better made without the pressure of an imminent problem.

It is imperative that the caregiver and the care recipient discuss the future openly and honestly. Emotions and plans should be discussed before an emergency arises. In fact, the recipient is often relieved when decisions about the future have been made. It is more often the caregiver who is reluctant to openly discuss these important issues.

It is not uncommon, however, for the older person living at home both to refuse to admit that care is needed and to refuse any alternatives. The fact is that it is usually difficult for any of us to accept help. For many of us, the notion of needing assistance has, since childhood, been equated with weakness. Likewise, needing help can raise fears of helplessness. Old age is a time when we will probably need to accept help. The closer that time comes, the more difficult and frightening it can be. For some people, the prospect of accepting help is so demeaning or frightening that they simply deny the reality of their situations.

In such cases, consultation with the care recipient's physician or a mental health professional may be helpful. Sometimes, a discussion with a professional about the stress of growing older is sufficient to bring about a more realistic view of the future. However, when a recipient refuses help and that refusal puts him in danger, professional help must be sought immediately. The recipient's physician or a local mental health facility can advise you on how to proceed.

If you are in a position of providing care to someone in his or her own home, be realistic about how much time and energy you have, especially given other demands on your time. If you are not able to give the person the care he or she needs, do not hesitate to investigate community services that might be available to help you.

The Caregiver's Home

Often caregivers, especially adult children, are faced with the decision of whether to have their elderly parent(s) live with them. The introduction posed some important questions to be asked before this decision is made. In this section, some of these questions will be further explored. While these questions are posed primarily to adult children, most of the issues have equal relevance to a spouse or partner who is considering whether or not his or her mate can be cared for in the home.

The first question to ask is often the most difficult. Is having your parent or mate at home with you something you really want to do or are you considering it only because you feel as though you should? Having an elderly parent move into your home can be very stressful, particularly if extensive caregiving will be part of your role. Be honest with yourself. Are you willing and able to have your parent live with you?

How will having a parent in your household affect your family? It is critical to discuss the possibility with your entire family. If you have children, how do they feel about it? Will they have to give up things such as their own bedrooms, which may cause future problems and resentment? What has their relationship been with the older person and how might this affect the family's adjustment?

If you are an adult child, what does your spouse or partner think about the situation? Who actually will be providing most of the care? Women generally provide most of the actual physical care of older people. If you are a son thinking of having his parent move in, will your wife be the one who will be expected to provide most of the care? What impact will this have on her daily life and how does she feel about it? The presence of another person, particularly a person who may need increasing amounts of care in the future, is a decision that affects the entire family.

Does your parent really want to live with you or are you pushing for this move? Remember, an environment that is a problem or concern for you may not be perceived as a problem by your parent. A move can be very traumatic for an older person, particularly if he or she will have to leave familiar and loved places and people. A move that places a parent in a better environment but away from everything familiar can leave the older person confused, isolated, and lonely.

Persons who have sensory impairments, especially vision problems, may be very frightened by leaving the familiar. If you have lived in the same place for a long time, it is easy to negotiate your way around even if you see very poorly. Sometimes an older person will refuse to move, not only because of fear of trying to get around in a new place but also because moving to a new home will force him or her to face increasing disability.

It is particularly important that you reflect on the nature of your relationship with your parent. How did you get along in the past? How do you get along now? Old age usually makes us "more of what we are." Your parent is not going to be any different when he or she comes to live with you than he or she was before—people do not change just because they grow old. If you and your parent have always had a relationship full of conflict and argument, chances are that will continue when your parent moves in with you. If your parent was a person who always had difficulty with his or her own children as teenagers, chances are that he or she is going to have difficulty adapting to your teen-aged children.

How did you and your parent resolve conflicts in the past? Do you have a history of discussing problems and reaching mutually satisfying resolutions, or are denial and withdrawal part of your pattern? There will be many changes for all persons involved, and change usually involves problem solving and compromise. If these areas have been problems for you in the past, the two of you may need to see a counselor for help in learning effective means of problem resolution.

Determining the way you feel about illness and disability is critical. Not everyone can tolerate working with a person who is ill or disabled. It may be that you can provide some care but not all of it. For example, you may not feel able to provide care for certain physical problems, such as a colostomy. This is not a reflection on the kind of person you are. It is simply a fact that we all have differing abilities. It is important for you to be honest with yourself as to what you can and cannot handle. While it may be painful to admit that you are not able to deal with your parent's particular illness, it is far better to acknowledge this than to later find yourself in a situation that is intolerable for both you and your parent.

Old age can mean disability and an increased need for care. Some illnesses, such as Alzheimer's disease, can destroy any semblance of what the person was like earlier in life and leave in its wake a stranger who needs almost constant care. If the past relationship with the parent was a good and positive one, you will have the memories of earlier good times to ease the current-day realities of caregiving. If the past relationship was filled with conflict, there will not be the solid foundation that a positive relationship might yield. Anger and resentment about caring for the person as well as old conflicts are more likely to surface under the stress of caregiving. If your parent gave up his or her home to move in with you, both of you may feel angry and resentful, trapped, and unable to "undo" the earlier decision.

What will the costs of caregiving be for you? The costs will be emotional and physical, as well as financial. Will you be able emotionally to face the increasing illness and disability of your loved one? What kind of care and how much care are you physically able to provide? If you have illnesses or disabilities, it is important to consider how these may limit your ability to provide care to your parent.

Caregiving often involves very hard physical labor, such as turning a person in bed or helping to get a person into and out of a bed, chair, or bathtub. Are there other family members who can help with these tasks? Although there may be community programs to help with some of these tasks, such personal care service is expensive and/or in short supply. Do not try to take on more than you can physically handle. If you become exhausted or hurt, who will be there to care for your parent or mate?

The financial cost of caregiving can be great. It is important for you to realistically assess how much the cost will be before moving your parent into your home. If you work outside the home, will you have to give up your job to care for your parent? There are programs that may help provide some financial assistance, such as Florida's Home Care for the Elderly program. But any of these assistance programs will not be enough to compensate for the loss of a job.

On average, how much does medical care for your parent cost and how much of it is, or will be, covered by insurance? Is your parent's insurance coverage transferable to where you are living? For example, some health maintenance organizations (HMOs) will only pay for local physicians and hospitals. Moving the care recipient outside an HMO's service area might eliminate coverage.

It is important to determine who may be able to help you carry the financial burden of caregiving. For example, to what degree can the care recipient contribute to the cost of care? Are there others, such as brothers and sisters, who may be able to help? Dealing with finances can often be one of the most sensitive areas among family members. While one would not expect to borrow money from someone outside the family without an agreement on terms of repayment, requesting a contract from a family member is seen as disloyal and distrustful. All too often, family members make verbal agreements about contributing to the cost of care, agreements that go by the wayside under the stress of other obligations.

Any agreement having to do with the sharing of caregiving responsibilities should be written and agreed to by all persons involved prior to having the recipient move into your home. Such agreements are very useful in regard to actual care activities, such as transportation to a physician and establishing temporary responsibility if you choose to go on vacation.

Certainly, this rule should include any agreements regarding financial concerns. Not only does this clarify responsibilities, it will also help avoid problems with any family member who might interfere with your, and the care recipient's, financial affairs. If there is any chance that the agreement may be challenged, you should consult an attorney.

Daily Caregiving: Issues and Challenges

CAREGIVING ISSUES OF SPOUSES AND PARTNERS

It can be both extremely rewarding and extremely painful to provide care for your mate. At times, caregiving can strengthen the bond between the two of you and deepen your commitment and intimacy. Caring for your loved one can give you a sense of pride and accomplishment that you have been able to meet the challenges necessary to allow the two of you to stay together.

At the same time, it can be almost unbearably painful to see someone you love become frail and increasingly disabled. A disease such as Alzheimer's can rob you of your relationship. The constant care and supervision required, the emotional and physical strain, and the isolation and financial burden of care may result in extreme and debilitating stress.

Most mates believe that they will "grow old together." When one grows to need care, the caregiver can expect to feel saddened, cheated of the plans that were made together, and sometimes resentful that life did not turn out the way it "should" have.

"Who will take care of me?" is a very real question for mates who are older and particularly for those who do not have children. Feelings of fear, anger, sadness, helplessness, and being overwhelmed can all be expected. You need to be very aware of your own physical condition and limitations so that you do not become ill. In addition, it is extremely important that you maintain contact with friends and relatives. Although you may be the primary caregiver, emotional support and relief provided by visits with friends and family is essential for your well-being.

CAREGIVING ISSUES OF ADULT CHILDREN

Adult children have special problems in dealing with aging family members. It is very difficult to see our family members age. We would like to think of our family—especially our parents—as they were when we were kids. It is often reassuring, although we know that it is not true, to think that our parents are still there waiting to pick us up when we fail or to give us help or advice when we falter.

It often comes as a shock when we realize that not only are they getting older, but so are we. We need to consider caregiver responsibilities; it is unrealistic to think that our parents will be there to take care of us when we will probably be caring for them.

This process is often mistakenly labeled "role reversal." That is, our parents become more like children while we become more like parents to them. The notion of role reversal is not truly accurate and may be seen as demeaning by older family members who believe that they are is capable of handling life as they always have.

In fact, what is really happening is called filial maturity. This refers to the point at which adult children reach the level of maturity where they can be depended upon by their parents or other family members. No longer do children look to their parents for care. Instead, the children have reached a stage where they can take care of their parents if needed.

Filial maturity is a normal stage in growth and most adult children go through this stage without awareness of it. Sometimes, however, problems arise as this process unfolds. Hurts and resentments over the course of our relationship with our parents remain strong even into our later years. In addition, it may become difficult to view our parents as they are now, and even more difficult to see their need for care.

For example, let us say that, of two daughters, the youngest always received the majority of the attention from her mother. As the mother ages, she asks the older daughter to take time off from work or family to run errands, take her to the doctor, and provide house cleaning help. The older daughter may harbor resentment from the past. She may believe that her younger sister should take more responsibility, since she received more attention and support from their mother. She may feel that she is being taken advantage of and she may be angry at their mother. Ultimately, she may find that she is unwilling to provide the care their mother needs.

Problems in achieving filial maturity can cause distress to both the adult child and the parent. Often, neither the child nor the parent feels comfortable and secure with the relationship, and neither is getting what each needs from the relationship.

Emotional Challenges of Caregiving

Caregivers usually try to provide the very best care possible to their loved ones and are very concerned when they experience emotions that are not "appropriate." Sometimes a caregiver may have the normal negative thoughts and feelings associated with caregiving discussed earlier, but may feel very guilty about them. The caregiver might try to make up for these negative feelings by overprotecting the care recipient and providing too much care, thus not allowing the older person to do what he or she is capable of doing.

Another problem can arise when the caregiver loves the care recipient too much. Sometimes people mistakenly interpret love as unconditional acceptance of the care recipient and his or her behavior, no matter what that behavior might be. In this case, the caregiver may accept being treated in a demeaning manner and might even allow him- or herself to be manipulated by the care recipient. Unfortunately, the acceptance of a care recipient's negative behavior may reinforce that behavior and lead to anger and resentment on the part of the caregiver.

Caregivers sometimes have a great deal of difficulty in distinguishing between normal negative feelings and thoughts and those that are so overwhelming that they may lead them to abuse or want to abuse their care recipients. If you find yourself hurting or dangerously neglecting the person you are caring for, or feel as if you want to do so, contact help immediately. In an emergency, call your local telephone crisis line, usually listed in the front of the telephone book. These telephone counselors are trained to listen without judging you and will direct you to the best source of help in your area.

TAKING CARE OF YOURSELF

As a caregiver, it is critical that you take care of yourself. The strains of caregiving cannot be underestimated. Caregivers often become isolated due to the demands of daily life. Although it may seem to take more energy than you feel you have, it is critical to keep in touch with friends, neighbors, and others who can help you maintain contact with the outside world. Everyone needs a break now and then. Sometimes, just talking with a friend on the telephone can leave you feeling refreshed.

All caregivers, no matter how dedicated and capable, will need help once in a while. There will be times when you become ill and cannot provide care. There will be times when the care needed is beyond your physical abilities. Be realistic about your capabilities—if you need help, ask for it. It is very important to have in mind the people you can call for help. Some people find it helpful to make a list of who they can call upon and in what circumstances. For example, who can go to the grocery store for you or pick up a prescription? Who would you call if the person you are caring for becomes violent? It is best to make this list early in the caregiving experience because you might feel overwhelmed and unable to think clearly in a crisis.

Make sure that you take care of your health. Physical exercise is essential. Exercise is not only good for your body, but is also an excellent way to reduce stress. You may believe that you get plenty of exercise through your caregiving responsibilities, but this exercise is usually not helpful to body conditioning nor is it relaxing. Although it may seem difficult to build into your schedule, regular exercise will give you both physical and mental benefits that exceed the amount of time spent on it.

Good eating habits are another way you can take care of yourself. Making sure that you eat a balanced diet is essential to your health and stamina. Often, caregivers do not allow themselves time to have a relaxing meal, trying, for example, to eat at the same time they are feeding the recipient. Taking time to eat a leisurely meal in a comfortable place is one way to care for yourself.

Be sure to build in time to do some of the things you enjoy. While it may not seem as if you have the time to do anything for yourself, constant worrying and caregiving will cause severe stress, perhaps leading to illness. Reading a book, going shopping, listening to music are all things that will help you rest your mind as well as your body. It is helpful to make a list of the things you enjoy doing, building one into your day, each day.

It is extremely important that we allow ourselves to become aware of how we feel and to ask ourselves what these feelings mean. For example, feeling irritable, tearful, and exhausted may mean it is time to take a break and be by yourself, to read a book or take a walk. If it is not possible to let go of caregiving responsibilities even for a short time, it may be time to contact service providers in your area to investigate the possibility of someone coming in to relieve you occasionally. Even the most devoted caregiver cannot provide care 24 hours a day, 7 days a week. To attempt to do so can lead to severe mental and physical exhaustion. You need to ask yourself, "If I get sick, who will be here to care for my loved one? What will happen to him or her?" Put in these terms, it becomes clear that it is critical to take the time to care for yourself. Remember, there are people who will help you give the best care possible to your loved one. You are not alone.

The Question of Institutionalization

Whether and when to place your loved one into a long-term care facility, such as a nursing home, is one of the most difficult questions to answer. The decision is based not only on your current situation, but also on beliefs and experiences from the past. We all have attitudes and beliefs about placing people in institutions. Many people believe that one should always take care of a family member regardless of the situation. Some people might have made a promise to a loved one in the past to never put that person in a "home." These beliefs, feelings, and experiences add to the difficulty of making such a decision.

In considering placement in a facility, there are two people to consider—the care recipient and the caregiver. Chapter 11 deals with the nursing home decision and the circumstances leading to institutionalization. Addressed here are some of the emotional issues that face caregivers in considering institutional placement.

Ideally, the person who is being cared for will have considered the question of long-term care and will have made his or her wishes known prior to a decision being made. Given the level of care that may one day be needed, and given the technological and medical advances that prolong life, it is unrealistic for anyone to extract a promise that he or she will never be placed in a nursing home.

If you have already given your care recipient such a promise, it is important to realize that you made such a promise without the information and experience you now have. The promise was made with the best intentions but without the facts on which to base such a decision. Now that you are in the caregiving situation, the promise may need to be reconsidered and alternative arrangements made.

In considering institutionalization, it is very important that you honestly assess your caregiving abilities. How is your physical health? Are you physically capable of continuing to provide the kind of care that is needed? What about your mental health? Are you depressed and do you face the future with dread? Is your depression leaving you too exhausted to provide the kind of care you want to provide? Do you have so much anger built up that it is difficult to continue caring for the person?

What about your family's health? If there are other persons involved, it is essential to assess the impact of caregiving on them. How much are they having to give up for you to continue your caregiving role? While you may feel an obligation to the care recipient, you also have an obligation to yourself and to the rest of your family. It is important to balance the needs of the person you care for with your own needs and the needs of your family.

Caregivers often ask themselves questions about how much is "owed" to one's spouse or parent. They often ask themselves, "Must I give up my life for my parent/partner?" or "What do others want me to do and what do I really think I can do?" There are no rules to help you answer these questions. If you find yourself struggling with these issues, it may be helpful to seek counseling to help sort out what is best for you and the care recipient.

Seeking Help

Caregiving, with all its strains and rewards, raises issues and questions that many people have not previously had to face. We often need outside help in determining past feelings and in discovering how they are influencing both our behavior and our decision-making in the present. Counseling is highly recommended to help you deal with the emotional issues of caregiving. Counseling helps us work through our old problems with our partners or parents and to let go of past resentments and hurts, and allow us to experience the best possible relationship we can.

WHERE TO GO FOR HELP

Many states, including Florida, have extensive laws licensing the mental health profession. When persons are licensed, it generally means that they have met a specific standard of knowledge and experience in their particular field. In looking for a counselor, you should seek someone who holds a license or who is working to meet the qualifications needed to get one. There are four types of licensed persons you may wish to consider: a licensed psychologist, a licensed clinical social worker, a licensed mental health counselor, or a licensed marriage and family therapist—the exact terms may vary from state to state. Whenever possible, it is best to work with a person who has had experience in working with older persons and their families. Since there is no specific state licensing procedure for this area of expertise, you should ask the counselor about his or her experience in working with older persons. Do not be shy about asking specific questions, such as "How long have you worked in the field of aging?" and "What degree or degrees do you have?" Counselors are accustomed to being asked these type of questions and should not be offended by them.

You may find a qualified counselor in several ways. It is often helpful to ask your physician for his or her recommendation, or to ask friends who have been in a similar situation. If your area has an Alzheimer's support group, someone in the group may be able to give you a list of counselors who have been helpful to others, even if your care recipient does not suffer from Alzheimer's. Your local Area Agency on Aging, too, may be helpful in recommending a qualified counselor. The Yellow Pages in the telephone book list mental health professionals, usually under headings "Psychologists," "Social Workers," "Psychotherapists," and "Marriage and Family Therapists." Counselors may operate in private or group practices or may work in an agency. Often, one of the best sources for finding a counselor is through your local community mental health center. Community mental health centers have special gerontology programs for older persons. Even if they are unable to provide the exact help that you need, they may be able to recommend someone who can.

Many insurance policies include mental health benefits, which will help defray the cost of counseling. The cost of these services is usually based on an hourly rate determined prior to treatment. Costs vary widely, depending on location, type of professional and whether the person or agency offers rates on a sliding scale based on ability to pay. Prior to making an appointment, be sure to ask what the cost is and if the person or agency will accept your insurance as payment.

People often are afraid to go to a counselor because of old beliefs that only "crazy" people seek mental health assistance. This myth is unfortunate because it prevents many people from getting the help they need. Caregivers are not the only ones who suffer from not getting needed help. Care recipients often do not receive counseling, which might help them deal with the fears, depression, and sense of loss that often accompany physical and mental illness. While it is often very frightening at first to go to a counselor, it can bring immense relief to talk with someone who understands your situation and who can help you reach a decision is to what is best for you and for the care recipient.

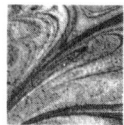

Profile

"*P*at" *is the 73-year-old wife of a retired minister. In 1972, she became a caregiver for her elderly mother, who suffered from a form of dementia. Pat cared for her mother for three years, contending with night wandering and her mother's fear of her own reflection in mirrors. "I finally put covers over every mirror in the house," she says.*

Pat's mother lived with Pat and her husband, "Joe," for three years until nursing home placement became necessary. She died in 1980 while Pat was traveling with her son to another part of the state for a brief visit with friends. It was the only trip Pat took in the eight years her mother was in her care. Pat has never forgiven herself for being out of town when her mother died.

In 1986, Joe, now 74, suffered the first of five disabling strokes. Through intensive rehabilitation, Joe is now able to get from his bed to a wheelchair and from a wheelchair to the toilet or shower. Pat must be there to assist him and to call for help should he fall.

"My husband was always the smart one, the leader," Pat says. "Now I'm the one having to take care of all the situations that arise."

Pat says that she is in good health despite a brush with cancer two years ago that required a colostomy. She will keep Joe at home "as long as he is conscious and aware of his surroundings and physically able to stay." Yet, when she learned that a friend's elderly mother was in declining health, she did not hesitate in suggesting that a nursing home might be the best alternative.

Pat and Joe have three children. Their eldest daughter lives in Hawaii. A son and daughter, both in their thirties, live within 50 miles.

Pat had come to rely on her son for moral support, but he recently married and became an overnight father to two small children from his wife's previous marriage. He has less time and energy now to devote to Pat's and Joe's daily crises.

Joe's companionship is what Pat misses the most. "We used to have a lot more conversation and we could confide in each other and talk," she says. Once a voracious reader, Joe now spends most of his time in front of the television set.

Many friends and coworkers have not seen Joe since his last major stroke. Pat said she believes that people are afraid to visit a person who is not as he or she once was. Joe's devoted secretary said that she did not want to see him in a diminished capacity; she wants to remember him as he was.

Pat manages to get out to visit friends, until recently bringing in a sitter for Joe. The last two times she has gone out, she has left him unattended. On a recent day, she had just returned from a 70th birthday party for a longtime friend. "When you live to be 70, you've lived a full life," she says.

When pressed for advice, Pat declines. "Everybody is different," she says. "I'm not trained for this. I just do the best that I can." But Pat says that she has learned to try to think about things from Joe's perspective. Because he is nervous, she takes special care not to make sudden, loud noises. She is ever-so-careful when she drives with him in the car—usually to the doctor's office or a rehabilitation clinic.

The simple act of getting in and out of the car is a major ordeal for Joe—and for her. "Cars are not made for handicapped people," she says. Joe has fallen more than once despite Pat's best efforts. Their biggest fights generally center on Pat's handling of a caregiving chore, she says.

Pat says that she is fortunate. She knows that disability can bring out a person's worst qualities. Joe, she says, is usually the same sweet-tempered man he has been throughout their 49-year marriage. "I find a great deal of satisfaction in doing this for my husband," Pat says. "After all, he was so good at taking care of us."

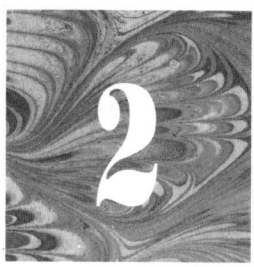

Legal Aspects of Caregiving

Tann Hunt, J.D.

She was middle-aged, widowed with two children, and living in the North. Her parents in Florida were ill; her 10 brothers and sisters had spouses and jobs that prevented them from providing care. She sold her house, packed up her children, and returned to Florida. Her parents' house, shabby when she was growing up, was now in serious disrepair, with no facilities for two people in wheelchairs.

On her parents' farmland, next to the old homestead, she built a large and modern home with room enough for her children and her parents. It took all the money from the sale of her "up north" home, but the new home had all the special features her elderly parents needed. Within a year, her mother died and her father had a severe stroke.

Suddenly the brothers and sisters found time—time to point out that the house had been built on the parents' land, to which the caregiving daughter did not hold title. Enter the lawyers.

In examining the special legal provisions available to caregivers and their older loved ones, it is clear that the best time to consult an attorney is at the outset of the caregiving relationship. It is important to remember that older persons do not belong in a legal geriatric ghetto. An older person may find that his or her legal needs can be met through some of the protections described in this chapter and still be part of the larger legal picture. Sell the house? Get advice from a real estate attorney. Slip on a wet spot at the grocery and break a bone? Consult a personal injury lawyer.

The flip side of this equation is that the caregiver may be in need of special legal protections. All too often we hear of caregivers who spend years providing for an elderly and, perhaps, difficult parent, only to find that all the money has been left to an uncaring—and uncaregiving—sibling.

Every family situation is different. Each caregiver has his or her special relationship with the care recipient and other family members and friends. There are no hard and fast rules that dictate that a particular legal action needs to be taken to protect the parties.

There are families in which a person's word is better than any legal document or court order. There are families that would be truly shocked by the suggestion that anyone's "rights" need to be protected through consultation with a lawyer or the signing of legal documents. But, as we all know, there are those families in which distrust, jealousy, and ill will have been part of the family structure from the day the marriage vows were spoken. The distrust and ill will were passed on to the children as if they were genetic traits.

There are also those families in which there is a legacy of love and trust. But even these special relationships can be eroded by the ravages of disease. "He was never like that!" you may say. All too true, but he is "like that" now, and now is the reality with which you have to deal. The loving, humorous gentleman has become the snarling, suspicious solitary.

It goes both ways. The sweet baby, catered to by all, grows up believing that he is entitled to whatever he wants, regardless of others' rights. He was an only child, spoiled by his parents. Rarely was he made to face the consequences of his actions. When things went badly because of his poor choices or inadequate effort, it was always someone else's fault. His parents worked hard, saving as much as they could, doing without, to better be able to care for themselves in their old age and not be a "burden" on their son.

Cancer claimed his father long before he ever had an opportunity to use the hard-saved funds. His mother continued to work, storing away money against the future. A large, old-fashioned home downtown became worth more and more as the restoration of such large places became fashionable. The property was sold, the taxes paid, and the money carefully put into certificates of deposit—in both the mother's name and the son's. "It's just for convenience, Mother," he said.

By the time his mother discovered that her son had left town, her money was gone. All of those carefully saved dollars, including the funds from the sale of the family home, were gone—to drugs and to bad "investments." Had the relatives who are now responsible for the mother's caregiving had a say in the arrangements, legal protections could have been built in for her. Not only did his mother never believe that her son would steal, she really never understood that she had helped set up a procedure that made it all so easy for him.

The laws of Florida provide many avenues to protect both the caregiver and the care recipient, but no chapter, no book can be a complete guide to these laws. Every situation is different. The best that this chapter can do is to alert you to the fact that there are legal avenues you may wish to pursue and to assist you in formulating intelligent, productive questions for your lawyer.

Back to Basics

An experienced caregiver, learning that this chapter was under preparation, said firmly, "Get the basics."

Regardless of the caregiver's level of involvement, the basic information is essential. If you are just helping, you need to know. If you are taking over, you need to know. If you are the personal representative after death, you need to know.

And what are the basics?

- Health insurance policies
- Nursing home care policies
- Car insurance policies
- Homeowners (or renters) policies
- Social Security numbers (the care recipient's and his or her spouse's)
- Pensions (military, state or private)
- Bank account numbers (checking and saving)
- Location of safe deposit box
- Other investments (stocks, bonds, certificates of deposit (CDs))
- Real estate property descriptions
- Homestead exemption entitlements
- Medical records, especially regarding adverse reactions to medications
- A complete list of medications
- A complete list of treating doctors
- Outstanding debts

- Location of the will
- Funeral and burial arrangements
- Existence of a living will, if any

THE "A-WORD"

Nobody wants to talk about it. In most peoples' minds it is worse than cancer. It makes a heart attack sound like a vacation. It is Alzheimer's.

Should someone for whom you are a potential caregiver be diagnosed as having Alzheimer's, run—do not walk—to the nearest competent attorney. This is the time when a durable power of attorney must be executed, before the disease has taken its toll, leaving the family with guardianship as the sole protection for the victim. While Alzheimer's is in its earliest stages, the victim is legally competent and able to execute the durable power of attorney. This can save money and misery after the ravages of the disease are felt. This also is the time for execution of a will.

THE WILL

Financial planners, lawyers, and interfering relatives say, quite accurately, that everyone should have a will. Some feel that it may be more important for a young couple with small children to have a will, providing for the children's financial and personal well being, than it is for an older person. Still, when one becomes a care recipient, a will is crucial.

Any will worth having is one that is drawn by an attorney, not something written out in longhand based on material copied from a how-to book. Wills can be as complicated or as simple as the facts, properties, and personalities require. For some, avoiding probate is a major consideration. There are ways to do it; they may or may not be worth the time and expense. Whether probate avoidance is appropriate for you or your loved one is best determined by an attorney.

For many people, the issue of concern is not the distribution of the monetary proceeds of the estate. It may be understood that they will be divided equally among the children. Certain funds may be left to charity, with others left in trust for children or grandchildren. What matters to many who are involved in making a will is the allocation of personal possessions that mean so much to the will maker and, hopefully, to those who will receive them.

The Florida legislature has devised a method for setting out how these personal items—not real estate, not money—are to be allotted. To accomplish this, the attorney who prepares the will must include a "separate writing" provision saying that items of personal property are being disposed of in a separate document. The provision also says that if the will maker has determined who gets what in a written document signed, dated, and separate from the will, those determinations will be honored.

The wonderful feature about this separate writing provision is that it allows the will maker to have frequent changes of mind without accruing additional legal expense. One week the second-best china goes to the elder daughter. The next week the second-best china goes to the younger daughter and the set of best china is divided equally. The antique sewing table goes to the nice neighbor next door, the small pearl earrings to a younger sister. The opportunities for rearranging items and people is endless and inexpensive. All the law requires is that the separate writing be dated and signed for it to be effective.

There are certain "technicalities" that must be addressed, whether one executes a will on one's own—still not a good idea—or with the aid of an attorney. Certainly working with an attorney on a will is a far better procedure, for a person's particular situation may be such that special provisions need to be included, of which the will maker might be unaware.

The ground rules are:

1) The will must be written. That which is simply spoken or even videotaped is not sufficient to do the work of a will. Some attorneys, especially where the soundness of the will maker's mind is at question, will videotape the will signing.

2) The will maker, known legally as the testator, must be of sound mind at the time the will is made. Law books are full of cases in which it is determined what constitutes sufficient soundmindedness for the making of a will. Again, this is the advantage of having a competent, ethical attorney to help you or a family member in drawing up a will. This is why it is especially important that a person who receives an Alzheimer's diagnosis immediately make a will while there can be no valid challenges to the will maker's mental state.

3) The will must be signed by the testator at the end and in the presence of two witnesses. A well-drawn will has a signature line or a place for initials at the bottom of each page, and each page is clearly designated—for example, "Page 2 of 10."

4) The will must be signed in the presence of the testator by two people who saw the testator sign the will. Frequently, attorneys will

provide three witnesses, recognizing that in some states three witnesses are required and thus protecting the will should the maker move to one of those states. A careful attorney will require that the will be notarized as well as witnessed.

For the will to be valid, the witnesses do not need to know, and, in fact, should not know, what the will contains. They are not witnessing the contents of the will; they are witnessing its signing. What they should be witness to is a statement by the will maker that she has read the will, that it says what she told the attorney she wanted it to say, and that she is freely and voluntarily signing it because it represents her wishes. The details of this are, of course, none of the witnesses' business.

A will can be undone by shredding it, burning it, or in some other way removing it physically from this world. But a destroyed or partially destroyed will means legal limbo. It is far more efficient for a will maker to replace the old will with a new one. The creation of a new will represents the present intent of the testator and, by its creation, replaces the old will. It is also possible to change a will by way of a codicil, a sort of "P.S." Matters of this nature are best left to an attorney.

Florida has specific restrictions and provisions regarding homestead property and surviving spouses. These are outside the scope of this chapter, but the reader should be aware of them. The various forms of joint ownership should be evaluated with an attorney as to what is most suitable for a particular person's situation. It is especially important that these effects be reviewed with an attorney. What seems a simple way to handle money matters and "avoid probate" can turn into a legal jungle, either before or after death. The cliche "penny wise, pound foolish" may have been created to describe the person who wishes to avoid paying an attorney to set up will and to give advice on the handling of various ownerships. The person whose bank account was cleaned out by a once trusted co-owner has not saved money. A person whose heirs must resort to the court to fight over the remainder in a joint ownership account has not saved money for the family.

WHOSE LAWYER IS SHE ANYWAY?

A lawyer has an ethical duty to represent his or her client. This duty creates boundaries for the lawyer and his or her relationship with the caregiver and other family members.

The caregiver may want an attorney to assist the care recipient in drawing up a will that provides for the caregiver. If the care recipient wants to do this, all is well. If, however, the care recipient wants to leave all of his worldly goods to other relatives, friends, or charity, the lawyer is obligated to create a will reflective of those wishes—unless he or she has reason to believe that the care recipient is incompetent and not in a sound mental state.

An ethical lawyer will meet privately with his or her client to ensure that the will says what the client wants it to say—not what the family members want to hear. Confidentiality also protects wills from later challenges.

PRENUPTIAL AGREEMENTS

When an older couple marries, their grown children may rejoice—or they may develop anxiety over the fact that "their" inheritance may go to a stranger. Anxiety can be avoided if the bride and groom sign a prenuptial (pre-marriage) agreement. The legal requirements for prenuptial agreements are complicated. They are best prepared by an attorney. No one of any age should sign one without first consulting an attorney.

THE DURABLE POWER OF ATTORNEY

Florida law has a provision which, if used appropriately, can result in a substantial savings of legal effort and money. The durable power of attorney is a document by which a person spells out that another person will have the power to handle his or her business and personal affairs in the event he or she becomes incapacitated. (Older law uses the word "incompetent." Now, even judges use the terms interchangeably.) Usually, the grantor of this power of attorney names an alternate so that there will be a person there to fulfill the duties should the first person be unable or unwilling to do so.

The operative word in "durable power of attorney" is *durable*. A person can have a power of attorney for specific events, such as sale of a house or car, but the power vanishes when the event is complete. But the authority granted under a durable power of attorney remains effective until the donor dies, revokes the power, or is adjudged incompetent.

The durable power of attorney can be a most useful device for caregivers. But it can be an extremely dangerous device if it is left in effect after the grantor has reason to distrust or dislike the person to whom he or she has given the power.

The Florida Legislature in 1990 recognized that we live in a world in which family members may either be not close by or not necessarily of the spirit to carry out the responsibilities associated with a durable power of attorney. Previously, only family members could be granted durable power of attorney. Now a person may simply designate someone to be his attorney-in-fact. The new law says that the power of attorney may include authority for the attorney-in-fact to arrange for and consent to medical, therapeutical, and surgical procedures for the principal, including the administration of drugs.

In the event someone files a petition asking that the grantor of the power of attorney be adjudged incapacitated, the power is temporarily suspended. Should an emergency arise during the period of suspension, the holder of the power of attorney may petition the court for permission to exercise the power. It is hard to imagine a situation in which a declaration of incapacity would be sought after the creation of a power of attorney, unless tremendous conflicts between family are involved. The guardianship process is an expensive and emotionally difficult one best reserved for those extreme cases in which a power of attorney has been misplaced and abused.

For the wealthy, there is a living trust alternative to the durable power of attorney. This is quite complicated, requiring the service of an attorney who specializes in the field.

GUARDIANSHIP

Guardianship traditionally has been regarded as an expensive and awkward procedure. Due to changes in the law enacted in the late 1980s, it is now even more so.

Because unscrupulous people have used the Florida guardianship laws to take advantage of the sick and the confused, the legislature has recently enacted laws which provide for far greater court supervision than ever existed before. The concept of detailed court supervision to protect incapacitated persons is fine in principle and may, in some cases, be well worth the time and effort required for the protection it provides. For the average family with the average amount of emotional difficulties, greed, and ill will, however, guardianship is simply an extra burden draining whatever reservoirs of good will might be left. It is too soon to evaluate the actual value of the new laws.

Compared to the durable power of attorney, guardianship is expensive to put into place and demanding in the detail required of annual plans and reports. In addition to being time consuming and expensive, in the majority of cases it is humiliating and heartbreaking.

Few people go from competency on one day to incapacity the next.

The line between the two is often blurred, with the older person moving back and forth between a "normal" or "more normal" state and true incompetency. Therefore, a determination has to be made as to whether the person has crossed the line sufficiently to justify the removal of his or her rights.

There is no such thing as a "pretty" competency proceeding. The law is strict in the procedural methods required, specifying the persons qualified to render an opinion to the court as to the mental state of the care recipient. Notice is required to be given to the care recipient and to other relatives. If ever there was an open invitation to dig up old family hurts, this is it.

Guardians come in different categories. There are guardians of the property and guardians of the person. Most often they are one and the same, but the opportunity for there to be more than one provides yet another opportunity for family rancor.

In one family, the daughter was guardian of the person; her brother was guardian of the property. The daughter complained that the guardian of the property did not provide her with sufficient funds to take proper care of "the person." The son insisted that "the person" had deteriorated to such an extent that it really did not matter where he was and, therefore, a cheaper arrangement that would leave money for the inheritance would suffice.

THE MEDICAID MUDDLE

This complicated and unsettling area of the law is addressed in Chapter 12. Take warning: Medicaid law is now so confusing that lawyers are writing educational programs for other lawyers on the subject. Medicaid law—like aging itself—is not for sissies.

THE HEALTH CARE SURROGATE

The Florida Legislature has created an alternative to the guardianship process by which an adult may, prior to any incapacity, designate a surrogate to later make health care decisions on his or her behalf. A person designated as a health care surrogate must be notified of that designation and indicate his or her consent in writing. The designation, too, must be written and must be signed by the person naming the surrogate in the presence of two witnesses, one of whom must not be the spouse, a blood relative, an heir to his estate, or responsible for paying his or her health care costs.

When the question of competency to make a health care decision arises, two physicians, one of whom is the attending physician, must certify that the patient lacks capacity. The health care facility responsible for the patient then notifies the health care surrogate in writing that he or she is to assume the duties of surrogacy.

The surrogacy law also provides that if a patient has not designated a health care surrogate, or if the health care surrogate is unable or unwilling to act, the health care facility can arrange for someone to act as the health care surrogate. The legislature wisely prohibited any employee of the health care facility from serving as a health care surrogate for a patient.

THE LIVING WILL

Florida law recognizes the right of competent adults to make oral or written declarations instructing their physicians to provide, withhold, or withdraw life-prolonging procedures, or to designate another to make that treatment decision for them, in the event they are diagnosed as suffering from a terminal condition. The law sets out a suggested form for the living will, which appears at the end of this chapter.

This is not the sort of document that one makes and then carefully tucks away in a safe deposit box. A critically ill person is not going to be in a position to rush down to the bank, take the document out of the safe deposit box, and rush it back to the doctor, family, and friends. This document, once signed and witnessed, perhaps in multiple "originals," should be widely distributed. The primary physician should have one, any secondary physician regularly involved in care should have one, family members should have one, and, certainly, so should any person designated to make the decisions.

The Latest Word

The awkward provisions and gaps in the surrogate and living will laws were resolved by the Florida Supreme Court in the fall of 1990. Cutting through years of court cases, the Court acknowledged, "The decision to terminate artificial life-sustaining measures is being made over and over in nursing homes, hospitals, and private homes in this nation. It is being made painfully by loving family members, concerned guardians or surrogates, in conjunction with the advice of ethical and caring physicians or other health care providers. It is being made when the only alternative to a natural death is to artificially maintain a bare existence." Basing its decision on Florida's constitutional right to privacy, the Court held that a guardian, a formally named surrogate, or a close family member may carry out the wishes of an incompetent patient who has, in writing—or orally—expressed them before becoming incompetent.

Just as importantly, the Court held that there was "no legal distinction" between providing food and water artificially and any other artificial means of life support. Any can be terminated. Having said this, the Court did urge the citizens of Florida to express their wishes clearly. A living will remains the best way to do this.

The federal government now has a role in the matter. For nearly two years, all hospitals and nursing homes have been required to advise their new patients about preparing a living will. Far better for a person to make such serious decisions ahead of time at home or in a lawyer's office.

Advice for the Caregiver

In all of these matters, you will benefit from thinking as a law school attempts to make its students think: What can go wrong and how can it be prevented? It is out of such negative thinking that positive results may flow.

The Florida Bar, in conjunction with the Florida Bar Foundation and the Florida Justice Institute, periodically publishes the *Older Floridians Handbook*, a legal guidebook that addresses many concerns of the elderly. Requests for individual copies of the handbook should be submitted, in writing, to: Older Floridian's Handbook Project, The Florida Bar, 650 Apalachee Parkway, Tallahassee, Florida, 32399-2300.

If you are in need of a referral to an attorney who specializes in elder law, The Florida Bar Lawyer Referral Service may be able to assist you. The number is (904) 561-5844 or (800) 342-8011. Be sure to ask for referral to an attorney who serves on The Florida Bar's Section on the Elderly. Remember that the best referral will likely come from someone you know and trust who has personal knowledge of an attorney's abilities in this area.

DECLARATION

Declaration made this _____ day of _____, 19__.

I, _____, willfully and voluntarily make known my desire that my dying not be artificially prolonged under the circumstances set forth below, and I do hereby declare:

If at any time I have a terminal condition and if my attending or treating physician and another consulting physician have determined that there is no medical probability of my recovery from such condition, I direct that life-prolonging procedures be withheld or withdrawn when the application of such procedures would serve only to prolong artificially the process of dying, and that I be permitted to die naturally with only the administration of medication or the performance of any medical procedure deemed necessary to provide me with comfort care or to alleviate pain.

It is my intention that this declaration be honored by my family and physician as the final expression of my legal right to refuse medical or surgical treatment and to accept the consequences for such refusal.

In the event that I have been determined to be unable to provide express and informed consent regarding the withholding, withdrawal, or continuation of life-prolonging procedures, I wish to designate as my surrogate to carry out the provisions of this declaration:

Name: _____
Address: _____
_____ Zip Code: _____
Phone: _____

I understand the full import of this declaration and I am emotionally and mentally competent to make this declaration.

Additional Instructions (optional):

_____
_____
_____

(Signed)	(Signed)
(Witness)	(Witness)
(Address)	(Address)
(Phone)	(Phone)

DESIGNATION OF HEALTH CARE SURROGATE

Name: _____
               (Last)   (First)   (MI)

In the event that I have been determined to be incapacitated to provide informed consent for medical treatment and surgical and diagnostic procedures, I wish to designate as my surrogate for health care decisions:

Name: _____
Address: _____
_____ Zip Code: _____
Phone: _____

If my surrogate is unwilling or unable to perform his/her duties, I wish to designate as my alternate surrogate:

Name: _____
Address: _____
_____ Zip Code: _____
Phone: _____

I fully understand that this designation will permit my designee to make health care decisions and to provide, withhold, or withdraw consent on my behalf; to apply for public benefits to defray the cost of health care; and to authorize my admission to or transfer from a health care facility.

Additional instructions (optional): _____
_____
_____
_____

I further affirm that this designation is not being made as a condition of treatment or admission to a health care facility. I will notify and send a copy of this document to the following persons other than my surrogate, so they may know who my surrogate is.

Name: _____
Name: _____
Signed: _____
Date: _____
Witnesses: 1) _____
             2) _____

Legal Aspects

Ethical Aspects of Caregiving

Margaret Lynn Duggar, M.S., Ed.

Think back to when you were 16. You had been driving a car for some time and you knew that you were totally capable of doing anything. *Anything.* At some point, you no doubt had a difference of opinion with your parents as to whether you were going to be allowed to drive the family car to some important event. You knew that you could be trusted. Your parents said that it wasn't a matter of trust. You knew that it would be all right. Your parents said that it would not. Can you recall your frustration? Your anger?

It is possible that even more recently you have been on the parental side of this discussion—telling a teenager of your own that he or she cannot take the car somewhere. Or, possibly, you have been on the adult child side of this discussion, expressing to your aging parent why you believe that he or she can no longer drive. And that dialogue may have been the most frustrating and difficult of all, for both of you.

Issues of who decides when a family member should no longer drive and how those decisions are made strike at the heart of ethical aspects of caregiving. These are the questions with no easy answers—sometimes with no answers at all. Attention to the ethical aspects of those decisions not only assists caregivers in making the best possible decisions, but also relieves some of the tensions of caregiving.

Seven months after her husband died, Mrs. Shovall fell in her kitchen and broke her hip. It was almost two days before a neighbor noticed the newspapers on the front lawn and called the police.

When Mrs. Shovall's son and daughter arrived from out of town, they visited their mother in the hospital and became increasingly concerned about her disheveled appearance, her anxiety about the accident, and her general health. They began immediately to assess the home environment for its safety and their mother's ability to remain in her own home. They talked with the neighbors, with the physician, with her minister, with local congregate living facilities and nursing homes, and with community agencies. By the time Mrs. Shovall was released from the rehabilitation hospital, her children had agreed that she could no longer live in her home safely and had contacted a realtor to discuss putting her home on the market. Time was short, as both her son and daughter had full-time professional jobs in distant cities as well as family responsibilities.

On her second day home from the hospital, Mrs. Shovall sat with her two adult children and listened passively while they described the options for her future—each one well thought out and well organized. But each option was developed without Mrs. Shovall's involvement or knowledge. While the discussion was conducted as though Mrs. Shovall had a choice, it was clear to her that the most significant decision, that she could no longer remain in her home, had already been made by her children without her involvement. Now her decisions would be made within the narrow framework of choices that would simply carry out the initial decision.

What has really happened here? Mrs. Shovall has been deprived of her personal autonomy—she has lost her right to make the decisions that impact her life. That broken hip did not rob Mrs. Shovall of the capacity to make decisions about her life. It did render her temporarily dependent on two very competent, very caring adult children who, without consulting her, assumed responsibility for making her decisions. Their actions began a series of subsequent events for Mrs. Shovall that frequently occur when older adults suffer an assault on their autonomy: the rapid, downward spiral toward full physical, mental, and emotional dependency. Mrs. Shovall did agree to sell her home and move into a congregate living facility, and she did relinquish more and more decision-making authority to others, including her children. She became passive and depressed; soon she was dependent on others for assistance with bathing and selecting her food and paying her bills. Friends and loved ones spoke of how tragic that one fall and broken hip had been, of what a toll it had taken on her. No one realized that the beneficence of a caring family had rapidly turned to paternalism and that Mrs. Shovall had become the victim of her own caring children's attempts to make decisions they considered best for her. No one understood that the real tragedy was an ethical one and not a physical one.

Autonomy is self-determination, self-rule; it relates to the freedom of the individual to choose, to make his or her own decisions and determinations about life. *Paternalism* is "other- determination," "other-rule"; it relates to absence of the individual's ability to choose, to make his or her own decisions about life. In a paternalistic relationship, someone else—a family member, a social worker, a doctor, a nursing home staff member, or some other person—assumes the decision-making responsibility for the individual, similar to the way a parent would. Usually, the decisions are justified by having the person's "best interests" in mind. Nonetheless, the paternalistic behavior results in exercising control over the individual.

Typically, persons who make decisions for an older person in a paternalistic manner are well intentioned. Often, paternalism is defended as protecting the older person from dangers or injury, or even from bad decisions. Before being able ethically to justify paternalistic behaviors, a caregiver must weigh very carefully the actual probability and extent of harm. To justify making decisions for another person, the caregiver must be able "to show that the harm to be prevented or the benefit to be provided really outweighs the loss of autonomy and other benefits the patient or agent seeks in taking the risk(s) involved; that the intervention has a reasonable chance of producing the desired result; that it be a last resort; and that it employs the least restrictive and insulting means available" (Klinefelter, 1986). We each have the right to the dignity of risk and, unless a person's cognitive abilities are severely impaired, he or she has the right to involvement in every decision that affects his or her life.

Every caregiving situation presents changes in the relationships between the person receiving care and those who provide that care. The relationships are affected by the length of time of caregiving, by the shifts in the balance of power in the relationships, and by the responses both parties exhibit to the dependency of the person receiving care. What is important is not so much the changes in the relationships as the caregivers' behavioral responses to those changes. It is at this point that the subtle, and sometimes not so subtle, ethical aspects of caregiving come into play.

Caregiving naturally creates dependencies. We Americans abhor feeling dependent on anyone or anything. Actually, we delude ourselves if we believe that we are totally independent. We could not ride down any street without being dependent on those who pave that street, who orchestrate the traffic signals, who obey the speed limits, and who enforce the laws. Nonetheless, we believe in our Declaration of Independence and we will fight fiercely to maintain the independence.

This love of independence can result in the caregiving relationship being fraught with conflicts for all parties from the very beginning. Being dependent on others for activities you have always performed for yourself is a very difficult adjustment. Likewise, it is often troublesome for caregivers to acknowledge that the person they care about can no longer perform those functions himself or herself and that he or she requires assistance. Yet, it is a fact that the person requires help with some activities. The caution is to continue to involve the care recipient in decisions about when and where and how those services will be performed and not to generalize from those specific needs to take over other areas of decision making. It is essential not to allow the creation of a dependence in one area to diminish independent functioning in other areas, especially in decision making.

The major factor in determining an ethical balance in caregiving relationships is the role the older person plays in making decisions about his or her life. Unfortunately, whenever a person exhibits some frailty, either physical or mental, families often assume that the person is unable to perform other tasks as well. Or, when an older person who is totally competent makes a decision that family members find unacceptable, they may assume that he or she is losing mental competence. The fact may be that the person is genuinely deciding to do something that is different from anything he or she has ever done—a fully autonomous decision. Possibly, the person is merely making a bad decision—something that each of us has the right to do! The dilemma for older persons, particularly those with adult children, is that often they are expected to behave as they have always behaved, and certainly they are expected never to make mistakes.

Physical Limitations

Caregivers of persons with physical limitations can enhance those persons' autonomy in decision making by always involving them in decisions regarding when, where, how, and by whom services are to be performed. Caregivers usually are adding caregiving responsibilities to already full schedules, necessitating efficient decisions and actions. Time constraints often lead to assumptions instead of negotiated decisions and to shortcuts such as doing things for the individual that he or she could do independently if time was not a factor. In preserving autonomy in caregiving, faster is not necessarily better, and the most expedient methods can erode self-determination and individual self-worth.

In one case, Dad, who has lived alone for many years, is becoming increasingly unstable in his walking and is experiencing serious vision deterioration. Yet, he continues to insist on driving. Every time the family brings up the subject of concern about his ability to continue driving, Dad gets very angry and refuses to discuss it. The family is very concerned that Dad may have an accident and not only hurt himself but others as well. The family questions how they can respect Dad's personal autonomy when they feel that, although Dad is mentally sound, his decision in this matter is not a wise one.

There are a number of approaches that the family can use. First, they need to determine whether Dad's vision problem is affecting his driving. It is also important to realize why Dad would resist giving up his car. Acknowledging that he can no longer drive is one of the most significant decisions an older person makes. It involves relinquishing independence and power and admitting that frailty has caused you to permanently move into another dimension of life. Dad's resistance to giving up driving is very likely more related to his fear of dependence than his actual need to have his own transportation. It is the larger message regarding his capacity and independence that he is avoiding.

When the family tries to force Dad to confront the driving issue, Dad is probably responding from the perspective of the dependence he fears. At this point, it is useful to find intermediate solutions to the driving problem and to allow some time for the acceptance of the inevitable loss of independence. In fact, it is likely that Dad himself knows better than anyone else that his driving is problematic, but he has not yet been able to accept the enormity of the impact of that realization, nor has he determined what an acceptable solution would be. As an alternative to creating a tug-of-war over whether to give up the car, one option is for the family and Dad to work out temporary adjustments, because Dad is not a safe driver this week or this month. By taking an incremental approach, families can ease the transition by involving Dad in all decisions. Allowing a neutral party, such as your family physician or a trusted family friend, to take a lead in the discussion may prove helpful.

Many of the same approaches would be appropriate if Dad's health were declining and the issues revolved not around his driving, but rather around the handling of personal affairs, particularly those involving business and finances. Here again, the larger issue for Dad may be the acceptance that his physical condition would warrant him relinquishing his decision making to a family member or business partner. The significance is in the dependence on others for making decisions he has always made himself. If Dad asks a family member or other caregiver to assist him with his personal affairs, it is essential that that individual not make any decisions, even routine ones, or take any actions without Dad's involvement and authorization for as long as he is able. Of course, the mortgage and the utility bills need to be paid, but not without Dad's express knowledge and/or instruction to do so. Assuming responsibilities to "relieve Dad" would erode his autonomy, his trust, and his dignity. It would encroach on the ethical aspects of caregiving.

Critical personal decisions need to be made with the full participation and negotiation of all parties involved. Relevant issues to be jointly decided include: what and when to eat, when and how to bathe and dress, sleep schedules, participation in leisure activities, interaction with family and visitors, and medical decisions.

What do you do when the care recipient refuses to acknowledge his or her physical limitations and realistically adjust or adapt decisions and behaviors to them? Suppose the person's vision has deteriorated to the point that driving is no longer safe. What if his or her equilibrium is impaired and climbing the ladder to clean the gutters is now dangerous? What if the older person living alone has fallen in the home 11 times in one month? Those who care must respond. It would be uncaring and irresponsible not to do so. How does a caregiver create the dialogue to identify changes that need to take place and arrive at conclusions in an environment that enhances personal autonomy?

First, create the most positive setting, both in time and in place, for an honest, adult-to-adult dialogue. It may be useful to remember that none of us sees ourselves as we really are at any given time. Our self-image rarely catches up with current facts. Marketing experts, for example, say that many people see themselves as 15 years younger than they really are. Likewise, most older persons will not view themselves as frail or disabled. A good way to lead in to the discussion, then, is to establish an agreed-upon baseline, a Polaroid view of the current situation, and realistic projections for the immediate future, usually no more than two or three months. It is dangerous to assume that everyone, including the older person, views the "facts" of the current situation in the same way. It is essential to begin by getting each party to describe fully current conditions as they appear to him or her.

The next step is an honest discussion of options for addressing the needs that emerge from the current conditions. While it is useful to be creative, it is also essential to be realistic. Each approach needs to be considered for both its long- and short-term values. For some families, committing to provide all transportation should the older person relinquish his or her car would be a workable solution. For others, following through on such a commitment would cause continual stress and strife. Inviting the older person to relocate into the adult child's home works for some families, while for others it exacerbates relationship problems and creates additional tensions. In some cases, it is the older person who feels that the extended family under one roof is not appropriate for him or her. In others, it is the younger family members who find the living arrangements unsuitable. In every case, the dependency of the older person and his or her lessened power in the relationship can easily become the pivotal issue in undermining autonomy in the decision-making process.

It is useful to assess potentially problematic situations as early as possible. One clear barrier to the older person's autonomy is a lack of options. The number of options diminishes as the older person becomes increasingly frail or develops more complex problems. Early intervention typically involves more options and enhances autonomy in decision making.

The next step is to agree to try one or more options. To support the older person's autonomy to the maximum extent possible, it is useful to keep as many options available as possible. For example, if other living arrangements are tried, it is essential to keep the recipient's home available for his or her return. Many older persons who do recuperate in nursing homes have to reside there throughout the remainder of their lives because their homes have been sold and their household items disposed of.

Finally, it is helpful to expect change, to avoid the mind-set of permanent solutions. While some decisions may work effectively for two years or so, others may work for only two weeks. Families and other caregivers, needing stability for their own lives, often search for lasting solutions. Caregiving is a process, a constant renegotiation. At times the caregiver is negotiating with the recipient of care, at other times with the health care system, with insurance companies, with community service agencies, with other family members, and with the myriad other entities that become part of the caregiver's life.

Limitations in Decision-Making Abilities

If the care recipient has some loss of mental capacity, involving him or her in the decision-making becomes more difficult. There are options, however, depending on the type and the extent of impairment.

If the condition is one of increasing dementia or, perhaps, even a diagnosis of Alzheimer's disease, the dialogue and advance decisions need to be made while the person retains cognitive ability. In addition, persons with impairments frequently vacillate between "better" days and "worse" days, so there is the opportunity for at least limited decision making on some days. Often caregivers want to avoid any difficult or even unpleasant topics on "good" days, so they delay broaching the dialogue.

If the level of impairment is extensive, the activities of the older person will be severely limited as well. The types of decisions the older person becomes involved in making may also narrow. As overall capacity for decision making becomes diminished, typically the activities of daily living (bathing, dressing, eating, etc.) dominate the person's time and energy. It is essential to maintain his or her involvement in decisions revolving around those activities: what and when to eat, when to bathe, or what shirt (or which of two shirts shown to the person) to wear. Attempts should always be made to involve the person in major decisions, such as whether to have surgery or other medical treatments.

When loss of memory results in failure to keep up with financial obligations, it can be very difficult for caregivers to offer the older person opportunities for autonomy. A forgotten water or electricity bill may very well result in the cut-off of utilities. Caregivers must recognize that the event cannot be undone. However, it cannot be ignored either. As with any problem, the person involved should be notified of the error, and so should the older person. The caregiver's responsibility is to help see that the issue is raised and, when appropriate, to help generate preventive measures so that it does not reoccur. Suggestions would include using a third party such as a bank trust officer or other business entity to pay routine bills. The care recipient might assign certain bills to be paid by a third party while retaining some bills to pay himself. A possible alternative would be for the older person to retain bill-paying responsibilities, with all bills sent in care of the caregiver or a paid care manager, who would meet with the recipient on a regular basis to pay all bills received. The key in these situations is to make the person aware of what has happened and to help him or her generate prevention strategies. It is also important not to go overboard. Who among us has never forgotten to pay a bill on time, mail payments, etc.? Some caregivers may be ready to schedule an incompetency hearing when a much less radical strategy, such as the involvement of a third party, will provide a solution.

Sometimes, loss of memory comes and goes, leaving caregivers in a constant state of flux—one minute the older person is clear and functioning, but before long the confusion returns with a comment like, "Where am I?" "Whose house is this?" Caregivers must be able to recognize the good days and offer as many choices and options as possible during those times. When the bad days come around, the caregiver must again adjust and revise the level of choices provided. During low-functioning periods, caregivers might be confronted with demands for handling finances or other high-functioning activities. How can a caregiver respond? By looking for associated or related issues where choices and decisions can be made by the older person. For example, if the caregiver normally maintains the financial records, allow the individual to review them. On some days, the choice might be whether to renew a certificate of deposit. On other occasions, the involvement might be sitting at the kitchen table while checks are being written.

Very often, an individual other than a family member or friend will be involved in providing services to an older person. For example, a housekeeper may be employed to provide services on a fee-for-service basis. Perhaps a live-in has been hired. Depending upon the degree of the recipient's memory loss, a great deal of trust is extended to the paid employee. From the caregiver's point of view, there may be a need to intervene and oversee this employer-employee relationship to protect the older person. There are two important things for caregivers to remember in these situations: 1) take time to get to know the employee and assure them that they play an important role in the care of the older person; 2) make sure that you do not step in where you are not needed. The relationship is between the older person and the employee, and the older person should always be afforded the right to make choices and decisions about employee-employer arrangements. If you suspect that the employee is not fulfilling his or her responsibilities or has otherwise exploited the relationship, the first step should be to discuss the issue with the older person rather than going directly to the employee. There may be a logical answer to your suspicions. Remember that the relationship is between the employee and the older person and that your involvement should be invited rather than asserted.

People often refer to a frail, older person as "childlike" or returning to his or her childhood. This is particularly common when the older person has cognitive limitations. The statement can subtly express permission to treat the person as a parent would. Older persons with impairments are not "returning to their childhoods." They are adults who have a disability. Some of the behaviors resulting from that disability are similar to behaviors of young children, such as the inability to operate household appliances or a lack of bladder control. They are just that— similar behaviors. No one actually returns to another stage in development. It is appropriate for parents to make some decisions for children until the child learns to analyze and assess consequences. With the impaired older person, however, we must provide him or her every opportunity and support to participate to the fullest extent possible in decision making.

Caregivers typically take on increasing responsibilities that can become overwhelming, both physically and emotionally. It may seem that investing the time and energy to involve an older, impaired person in all the decisions that affect him or her adds too much to the caregiver's burden. The reality is that caregivers typically assume their responsibilities because they care so very much, because caring for loved ones is integral to their most basic values, and because they want the caregiving done in the right way. Respecting the personal autonomy of that older individual is the ethical approach to decision making for frail older persons. They must assume the maximum amount of involvement in and responsibility for their own care that their capabilities permit. While the life of the older person may be different during this period of dependencies, it is nonetheless the life they are living at this time—and, hopefully, living to its fullest.

References

Klinefelter, D.S. "Aging, Autonomy, and the Value of Life." *Ethical Aspects of Aging Policy.* Tallahassee, FL: Aging and Adult Services Program Office, Florida Department of Health and Rehabilitative Services, 1986.

Long-Distance Caregiving

Marian Bruin, A.C.S.W., B.C.D.

Susan is a business executive in her home state of Michigan and is the mother of two teenage sons. Ten years ago, her parents, Richard and Barbara, left Michigan and eagerly joined their friends in Clearwater.

Richard purchased a condominium while he was still practicing medicine, and he and Barbara agreed to reside there year-round after his retirement. With their friends nearby, it was a very pleasant retirement.

Nine months ago, Richard passed away unexpectedly. Susan flew down to Clearwater and spent three weeks with her mother. Barbara's friends visited often, and she was able to maintain the condominium until recently. Barbara then suffered a minor stroke, and Susan again flew down to be with her.

Barbara was eager to leave the hospital. With the help of the hospital discharge planner, Susan was able to set up in-home physical and speech therapy as well as home health services before she returned to Michigan. Her mother, being a "private person," was uncomfortable with having strangers in her home. She became suspicious and began accusing them of stealing from her. When she refused to allow one of the home health aides to enter her home, Susan was called in Michigan and told by an agency representative that the agency could no longer provide services. He suggested that she begin looking for a nursing home.

Susan knows that her mother would not agree to move to a nursing home, and she also knows that her mother would not agree to come back to Michigan and live with Susan's family. Susan spends hours on the phone every day, trying to calm her mother down and allay her fears.

Even though her supervisors sympathize with her situation, they have expressed concern over the numerous distractions. Every time the phone rings, Susan's heart skips a beat. She is plagued with fear and guilt.

In today's mobile society, most adult children and their aging parents move at some time or other. It is not uncommon to find older relatives living a great distance from family members involved in their care.

The stresses, frustrations and responsibilities involved in providing long-distance care for an older family member are different from those encountered when that relative lives in your home or in your community. Long-distance caregivers are unfamiliar with the programs, services and resources in the area where their relative lives. Consequently, they are dependent on others—friends, neighbors, and the religious community—who live where their older relatives reside, to provide information, help and assistance.

A crisis or a new or changing situation may cause you to become much more involved, whether or not you are ready to assume the responsibilities of providing long-distance care. Where once you were able to listen to your relative's own reports concerning his or her health situation and general state of affairs, you now might need to speak directly with the doctors and others concerned with their care.

Your caregiving efforts will vary depending on the circumstances. Regardless of the extent of your involvement, it is very important to be realistic about how much you can do. The greater your involvement, the greater the impact will be on other aspects of your life, and you should not hesitate to enlist the advice and support of other family members, friends, support groups, and the religious community. Professional counselors should also be considered to help you as the demands of long-distance caregiving increase. You will need to reassess your commitment at various times so that you don't feel locked into a situation that has become untenable.

In some situations, providing financial assistance may be the main contribution that you or other long-distance caregivers can provide. Money can be used wisely and creatively to encourage your family member to try a needed service, or to pay for repairs or adaptive devices and equipment that will make the home safer and increase independence.

For many reasons, most people avoid planning for the future, and the time when they will no longer be independent. Confronting the issues ahead of time can help you get a sense of your relative's own wishes, so that the decisions that need to be made in the future can be made in a manner consistent with his or her own desires and choices.

Fear, guilt and constant worry are well-known emotions experienced by those people whose frail, elderly family members live at some distance. Fortunately, there are some practical, effective and well thought out remedies for those long-distance caregivers, aimed at helping them answer the following questions:

- How can I get help in a crisis?
- What exactly does my family member need?
- What are the best services in the community to meet those needs?
- How will the services be paid for?
- How can I make sure that these essential services are provided without unnecessary delay?
- How can I make sure that all the service providers work together on behalf of my family member?
- What additional resources are important?

Private Care Management

A new group of health care professionals who provide private care management has recently emerged to help older people and their family members focus on and resolve these exact questions and issues. They are independent practitioners-specialists with advanced degrees in the fields of social work, nursing, psychology, gerontology, and rehabilitation. Because they work in the community where the older person resides, they are familiar with the full array of locally available medical, home health, residential, social, legal, and financial services required by older people.

A private care manager can be your eyes, ears, and legs, helping you and your elderly family members make the best possible decisions. While private care managers offer a wide range of services, the degree to which you utilize those services will depend on your individual circumstances. You may have the ability, willingness, and time to do many of these things on your own. Because private care managers charge for their services, you may need to be selective about the extent of their involvement.

Services provided by private care managers include the following.

ASSESSMENT

One of the first priorities for private care managers is conducting a comprehensive assessment of your relative's physical health, activities of daily living (ADL) skills, social supports, physical environment, emotional status, intellectual functioning, resources, strengths, needs, wishes, and desires. Information is gathered during a face-to-face interview, and significant others are contacted for additional pertinent information. The private care manager can speak with you on the telephone or prepare a written report which summarizes the findings, lists the alternatives available to meet the needs, and recommends courses of action.

PLANNING

Once the assessment is complete, an action plan is developed that specifies the resources, programs, services, and supports required to meet the needs identified. The plan usually specifies immediate actions to be taken as well as procedures to follow in the event of an emergency. The private care manager can help you determine how to use your time and energy most effectively, and should be available to help implement those parts of the plan that you or other people in your relative's support network are unable or unavailable to implement.

COORDINATION

Securing services and resources to meet your relative's needs can be an overwhelming task, even for caregivers living in the same location as their loved one. Private care managers are able to coordinate your relative's health care and social service needs by arranging for both privately and publicly funded services and programs.

Because care managers are professionals, a quicker response to inquiries is usually received from doctors, hospital personnel, and other service providers. Publicly funded programs and services frequently have changing eligibility requirements and long waiting lists, and it sometimes takes an expert, with contacts in the field, to negotiate the bureaucracy and cut red tape. A private care manager can work with your relative's friends and neighbors in an effort to secure assistance and support. If you are spending significant time and money on calling service providers in another state, it may be more cost-effective to use a private care manager.

Many long-distance caregivers spend vast amounts on plane fares only to be exasperated over getting so little accomplished during their stays. A private care manager can fill out applications to receive services, accompany or arrange for your relative to be accompanied to scheduled doctors appointments, and attend meetings concerning your loved one. Regular telephone contact and periodic professional visits with your relative can also be scheduled, and you can be advised of newly identified needs as they occur.

MONITORING

Your relative's well-being, and the programs and services received, need to be monitored to ensure appropriateness and satisfaction. While it is true that many people receive less than what they require, it also is the case that some receive (and pay for) more than they need. Because no amount of money paid for a service can guarantee that service's quality or appropriateness, it can be very helpful to have the oversight of a skilled and independent professional.

If your relative is alone at home and receiving home health services, you will want to know how reliable the people providing that service are. If your relative is living in a nursing home or adult congregate living facility, you will want to know that his or her needs aren't being neglected and that they are free from abuse. By scheduling periodic visits with your relative, the private care manager can evaluate the quality and effectiveness of services provided, and take immediate action to correct the situation.

ADVOCACY

Many people are unaware of their rights and entitlements. Others, who may be well aware, are unable to advocate for themselves. In some cases, it requires not only a knowledge of the health care and social service system, but also a set of well-refined communication skills to secure and/or ensure quality treatment, benefits, and services. A private care manager can also advocate on behalf of your relative to preserve his/her well-being and dignity.

Locating a Private Care Manager

Currently, there is no state or professional licensure available for geriatric care managers, however, credentialing efforts are well underway through several of the professional care management organizations. Until such credentialing is available, you should be prepared to ask the following questions to determine whether the professionals you screen will be able to meet your family's needs:

- Is the person licensed by the state or certified by a national professional organization (i.e.,. a state board of nursing or social work)? Private care managers should be willing to show you copies of current licenses and certifications.
- What are the person's qualifications? How many years has he or she been providing care management services?
- Does the person carry professional liability insurance that covers care management services?
- Does the person provide care management on a full or part-time basis?
- Will the person be available in an emergency situation (i.e., after 5 p.m. and on weekends)?
- Does the person provide alternative coverage during times when he or she is not available?
- Is written information available that describes the full range of care management services that can be provided?
- Is a clearly written fee schedule available which specifies all charges?
- Is a letter of agreement or contract used which specifies the services to be provided?
- How knowledgeable is the person in the areas of both publicly and privately funded services?
- Does the person provide other direct services (i.e., home health services; transportation services; financial management services)? If so, what kind of checks exist to monitor any potential conflict of interest?
- Can the person arrange for you to speak with one or more of his or her other clients?

Private care management generally is not covered by private insurance. Rates range from $60–$120 per hour and in most cases, time spent on phone calls, professional visits, attendance at meetings, preparation of written reports, correspondence, and travel time are logged and billed.

The National Association of Professional Geriatric Care Managers (NAPGCM) provides a list of professionals across the country who may be able to assist you. The organization is located at 655 Alvernon Way, Suite 108, Tucson, AZ, 85711, telephone (602) 881-8008.

Providing Long-Distance Care Management Yourself

Ernest, a retired salesman, lives in New Jersey on a fixed income. He has been providing care for his wife, Frances, who has a mild case of Parkinson's disease. His parents retired to Naples many years ago, where they purchased a mobile home. They, too, lived on a fixed income. Five years ago, Ernest's mother died, and despite his pleas for his father, Jimmy, to come back to New Jersey to live, he refused the offer. Jimmy did not want to leave his modest home, his friends, or his church.

Several weeks ago, Ernest received an alarming call from Jimmy's next door neighbor, who had been helping him by dropping off groceries on a weekly basis. The neighbor said that it had been some time since he had been inside Jimmy's home, and on that particular day, he entered the home to find it in terrible shape. He said there was an unpleasant odor, which he assumed was caused by an air conditioning problem, and he noticed stacks of unopened mail lying on the dining room table. Jimmy clearly was not taking care of himself, but he denied that he was experiencing any problems.

The neighbor made it clear to Ernest that other than helping to resolve the air conditioning problem, he did not want to be involved in providing additional assistance to Jimmy. He suggested that Ernest take immediate steps to place his father in a nursing home, hire a home health service, or bring him back to New Jersey to live. Realizing that neither he nor his dad could afford the costs of on-going home health services, and that nursing home care would wipe out what little savings his father had, Ernest now is spending a considerable amount of time and money trying to keep an already bad situation from becoming worse.

Even though Ernest wants to, he is afraid to ask his father to move back to New Jersey, where he could provide care.

Becoming a provider and manager of care is not an easy task, particularly when the distance between you and your loved one is great. Whether or not finances are of great concern, it should be noted that the government does provide a host of programs and services to older people with limited incomes and, in some cases, limited assets. These programs and services are thoroughly discussed in Chapter 12. Competition for these services is great, and many programs and services have long waiting lists.

Unfortunately, a person's ability to receive many of the entitlements and other required services is directly related to the persistence of the caregiver and the intensity of the advocacy efforts required.

PROBLEM SOLVING AND DECISION-MAKING

One of the greatest difficulties of long-distance caregiving is that of being asked to solve problems and make decisions for someone who, until recently, was very much in control and self-sufficient. Many people in need of assistance will fight fiercely to maintain their independence. Sadly, as their mental acuity lessens, the easier it may be manage their care. At that point, the caregiver will have to rely on his or her own and others' knowledge of the care recipient's preferences, wishes, and desires. Bear in mind that the person whom you are trying to care for may well be his or her own best advocate.

The care recipient should be asked to participate in the decision-making process to the greatest extent possible. It will be important for you to understand your relative's emotional status and intellectual functioning so that you can determine the extent to which he or she can be meaningfully involved. When decisions that need to be made are made without the participation of the person who must live with the consequences, the results can be devastating.

GATHERING INFORMATION

If you are trying to provide or manage care from a distance, it will be essential for you to find out about the physical health and medical history of your family member, including current health problems. You will want a list of doctors', dentists', pharmacist's, and other health care providers' names, addresses and phone numbers.

You will need to know about allergies, medications, limitations, and adaptive devices or equipment that may be required. In order to make any decisions, you will need to determine the nature and degree of assistance needed by your family member to accomplish the activities of daily living, in the areas of physical self-maintenance and self-sufficiency. You will need a list of people who currently provide social and emotional support, so that you can coordinate care from a distance. You will want to know whether the environment is safe, sound, and secure so that you can make arrangements to correct any questionable situation and prevent future crises.

You will need information pertaining to health resources (Medicare, Medicaid, and private insurance), and income sources (Social Security, pensions, annuities and investments), to ensure that your loved one's bills are paid and that he or she is getting the benefits and entitlements that are due.

EXPLORING RESOURCES

Once you have gathered accurate information about your relative's health history and present status, you will need to explore the resources, programs and services in the community that can meet your relative's needs. There truly is no end to the number of services that may be required by your relative. A partial list may include:

- care management
- health and dental care
- emergency response
- financial assistance
- housing
- home health
- rehabilitation
- transportation
- socialization
- recreation
- nutrition
- home visiting
- telephone reassurance
- counseling
- spirituality
- housekeeping
- home maintenance.

To save time and energy, you may want to arrange appointments before your trip to your loved one's home state, and try to involve the care recipient by encouraging him or her to accompany you. It always is important to call more than one provider of a particular program or service, so that you can compare the services offered and the costs. In many areas, competition among service providers is great and rates may vary widely.

EVALUATING EACH ALTERNATIVE

After you explore the resources and alternatives that exist, you will need to evaluate which program or service would best meet your loved one's needs. You will want to ask the following questions to be able to arrive at a decision:

- Will the service/program accept your assessment, or will they conduct their own? If they make their own, will they come to your relative's home to administer it?
- Is there a waiting list for the service and, if so, how long is it?
- Are the staff who provide the service adequately trained and supervised? Do they have experience? Will they be reliable?
- What is the application procedure? Must your relative apply in person, or can you complete the application? What kind of documentation is required?
- How is the service paid for? Will Medicare/Medicaid or supplemental insurance cover any of the costs?
- How flexible are the services? If your loved one's needs change, will the services be discontinued?
- Is the organization that provides the service/program regulated by the state (i.e., licensed or accredited)? Is the staff bonded in the event of theft? Will they provide you with references from current clients?

ARRIVING AT AND IMPLEMENTING A DECISION

You will arrive at a decision by weighing the positives and negatives of each alternative, and choosing the one that will have the most positive and least negative effects and outcomes. You will want to evaluate each new program and service so that any problems can be corrected, and your relative and you feel that it is appropriate and meaningful. Agencies that provide health care and social services usually have a contact person who is familiar with the services your relative receives. By checking with your relative and the agency contact person, you can monitor how satisfactory the service is, and take the necessary steps to improve, correct, or terminate it.

CREATIVE PROBLEM SOLVING

If you manage care from a distance, you may need to find some creative ways to solve problems. You may want to subscribe to the newspaper in the community where your loved one lives, since new programs and services are often featured there. If your relative has a religious affiliation, you may want to contact his or her church or synagogue to find out what services they may offer and to apprise them of your interest and participation in your loved one's care and well-being. Frequently the spiritual needs of older people are ignored at that time in their lives when they should be intensified. The clergy often are willing to make home visits or to visit people residing in long-term care facilities to provide pastoral care. Members of a congregation frequently have well-developed telephone reassurance programs or "friendly visitor" services.

You may want to entertain the idea of getting a pet for your relative. An easy to care for pet, like a parakeet, might alleviate loneliness and brighten up the care recipient's days.

FINANCIAL AND LEGAL ISSUES

People work a lifetime, expecting to reap the benefits of their labor upon retirement. But soaring health care costs and the lack of a national long-term health care insurance program have impoverished millions of older people. Though the average person knows little about government benefits and entitlements programs, when long-term health care needs arise, one quickly discovers that Medicare will cover only a portion of the costs of much of the health care services required.

The state Medicaid program is intended to meet the long-term care needs of people whose income and resources are insufficient. Long-distance caregivers are advised to familiarize themselves with the eligibility requirements and to take the necessary steps early on to secure these benefits for eligible loved ones. In some areas of the state, it can take up to a nine months to process an application for Medicaid benefits. While benefits will be paid retroactively to the date of application if the application ultimately is approved, in many instances family members will have to cover expenses in the interim. This can pose a true financial hardship.

If your loved one hasn't already done so, you should contact an attorney who specializes in elder law about preparing a "living will," stating the care recipient's wishes about care in case of a life-threatening illness or injury. The attorney will likely suggest that other legal documents be executed, such as a durable power of attorney and the declaration of a health care surrogate, so that in the event of future incapacity, bills can be timely paid and decisions can be made on the care recipient's behalf without having to suffer the indignities of guardianship proceedings. Additional information pertaining to legal issues appears in Chapter 2.

OTHER ISSUES OF CONCERN

The care recipient may be in need of home health or companion services. That leads to the question of whether to hire someone privately or go through an agency to secure the services. Purchasing services through an agency saves paperwork, supervision, and time. But the cost may be significantly lower if you hire directly.

If you feel that your relative's needs will be best met by foregoing an agency, you will need to determine specifically what help is required and develop a job description. The job description can be turned into a contract that clarifies the duties and responsibilities of both the employer and the worker. This formalized agreement is essential if there is a dispute about hours of work, salary, or tasks to be performed. The contract and job description can be updated or revised as the need arises, and should be as specific as possible, to lessen the chances of confusion or disagreement. In addition to a description of the duties to be performed and the salary, you may want to include in the contract the terms of payment, fringe benefits (i.e., transportation fees, or meals provided), unacceptable behavior, and termination procedures.

The best way to hire a responsible person to provide in-home services to your loved one is through a recommendation from a friend, neighbor, or other person whom you trust. In Florida, the local Elder Helplines maintain a "sitters list" that identifies nursing assistants and homemakers who have gone through Department of Law Enforcement and abuse registry background checks. The care recipient's church or synagogue or a community organization that currently provides services also may be important resources.

If none of these methods work, then you may want to try advertising in the "Help Wanted" classified section of the community newspaper or in newsletters distributed by churches or social service organizations. The ad should include the number of hours needed, a very brief description of duties, a telephone number, and a time to call. Preferences such as non-smoker and the wage you are offering also should be mentioned.

You will not need to do a personal interview with everyone who responds to your ad. When respondents call, you should describe the job in greater detail as well as the expectations and wage range you are offering. It is important to know why they are interested in the job, and if they have previous experience.

If you identify individuals that appear to be qualified, schedule a specific time for a personal interview. Prior to the interview, you and, if possible, the care recipient should prepare a list of questions including:

- How do you feel about caring for an elderly or disabled person?
- Why have you chosen this kind of work?
- Do you have any physical or emotional problems which might affect your ability to work?
- How do you feel about cooking and eating what someone else wants?
- How would you handle a person who is angry?
- What makes you uncomfortable or angry?
- Do you have any religious convictions that might interfere with providing services?
- What is your attitude towards smoking, drinking, and/or using drugs?
- What commitment are you willing to make to staying on this job? Would you consider an initial "trial" period.
- Can you provide two work-related and one personal reference?

During the interview, have the job description and contract ready for the applicant to review and ask if there is anything in the job description that he or she would not do. Make note of whether the person arrived on time for the interview, whether his or her appearance and grooming was acceptable and his or her and your own comfort level.

If the applicant is clearly unsuited for the position, you can be noncommittal about future contact. Before ending the interview, remind any suitable applicant that you will be checking references before making any decision. *Never hire someone without first checking references!*

Among other things, you should ask previous employers about the duration and context of employment, the job applicant's reliability and trustworthiness and the quality of the relationship between the care recipient and the applicant. Most important, ask why employment was terminated and whether the employer would hire the applicant again if help of that nature were required.

Always conduct an abuse registry and criminal background check. Additional information is available in Chapter 14.

A signed copy of the contract should be given to the person who accepts the job prior to their starting. If you pay $50 or more per quarter of the year to an employee—and chances are that you will—you must withhold for Social Security benefits and make quarterly payments to the Internal Revenue Service. If you fail to do so, you may face prosecution by the federal government. Only if the person you hire meets the strict government definition of "self-employed" may you forego withholding.

Because weekly or bi-weekly paychecks may vary from one pay period to the next depending on hours worked, bookkeeping may become troublesome. It is essential tht accurate records be maintained.

You should check with the care recipient's homeowners' insurance agent about the extent of his or her liability coverage as it applies to an employee. For tax purposes, you should determine whether payments made to the employee will qualify as a medical deduction. Because of possible legal and financial problems associated with paying in cash instead of by check, you should be prepared to use receipt forms or other proof of payment to the worker.

Once strangers begin coming into your relative's home to provide care, you may want to remove anything of significant financial or sentimental value and store it in a safe place. It is very important to develop an inventory of belongings, especially if your loved one has impaired communication skills and is unable to advocate on his or her own behalf. It also is wise to make a list of all credit cards the care recipient may have, including the account numbers. This will enable you to cancel them in the event that they are lost or stolen or in the event that bills begin to appear that list charges you know your relative did not incur.

Bringing your loved one into your home

You may be in a situation where you must, for the sake of your own sanity, bring your family member to your home to live or to a residential facility in your community. You may do so because you are confident in your own ability to provide care, you are more familiar with services available in your own community, or because you wouldn't have peace of mind with your existing long-distance caregiving relationship.

Before making a move—and assuming that your loved one concurs with the decision or is unable to make the decision for himself—you should seek support and assistance from other family members, friends, your religious community, local support groups, and/or professional counselors. If you make the decision to become full-time caregiver, don't isolate yourself from the outside world. Help is available, although it will not always be easy to find. Above all else, *remember to take care of the caregiver.*

Successful Communication

Dawn Pollock and Judith Altholz, Ph.D.

Is what you heard what I thought I said?

Providing care for an older person is a generous and giving expression of concern and love. It also can be a difficult emotional experience for both the caregiver and the care recipient.

Good communication is an essential part of a successful caregiving relationship. The sensory changes that accompany aging can diminish our ability to communicate in social and in personal activities. While some people seem to adjust by planning ahead or compensating, others become frightened or try to ignore the changes. Frustration and stress can limit communication, making it more difficult to understand each other than it would ordinarily be. Communication can also be affected by existing conflict between the caregiver and the care receiver or by conflict that comes as a result of the changing roles involved in the caregiving relationship.

The foundation for successful communication is understanding. The more clearly we understand each other, the more successfully we can communicate. With some imagination, a little flexibility, and a degree of planning, good communication can continue in spite of the changes and limitations that may accompany aging.

This chapter will explore ways to maintain communication between the caregiver and the care recipient and will suggest techniques to help compensate for the limiting effects of aging, illness, and the loss of sensory ability.

Good communication is valuable because it can help to:

- identify changes in either physical condition or behavior
- maintain an older person's dignity
- continue a sharing relationship between the caregiver and care recipient
- enhance the effectiveness of day-to-day care
- solve problems that may arise
- improve treatment by involving the care recipient in as many of the decisions about care as possible
- maintain social and interpersonal contacts.

Some degree of change in our intellectual abilities and in our ability to see, hear, taste, smell, and touch are part of the normal aging process, which takes place at varying rates for all of us. As our medical knowledge of the aging process increases, it is easier to identify why various changes occur. Diminished capacity, which even recently has been attributed entirely to the aging process, may also be caused by disease, nutritional deficiencies, or medications. It is important for the older person to have regular medical checkups and hearing and vision tests, and for their physician to be aware of all prescription and over-the-counter medications the person is taking.

When changes related to aging are understood and techniques for compensation are learned, a great deal can be done to enhance communication and set realistic expectations for both the caregiver and the care recipient. Hopefully, we may also be more tolerant of limitations and less likely to stereotype or label a person as failing, confused, or senile. We may also be more likely to use hearing aids and other prosthetics with greater comfort.

Many methods have been devised to maintain or improve communication; adjustments can be made in behavior, the environment, or by using mechanical aids. For example, behavioral changes include learning to face the older person when you speak and allowing more time for an older person to express themselves. Environmental changes that can help communication include labeling medications in large bold print or painting stair edges with strongly contrasting colors. Finally, mechanical devices such as hearing aids, amplifiers, talking books, special telephones, and other items can also help to compensate for sensory loss or help orient a person who is confused.

There are several ways you can be a supportive communicator:

- maintain eye contact
- use active listening and attentive facial expressions
- reflect or restate what the person has said, to help clarify meaning to see if you have understood correctly
- sit near the person and try to position yourself on the same level
- wait patiently for responses
- if appropriate, touch the person you are talking with
- empathize
- be honest
- omit distractions and background noises
- slow down if it helps the person understand
- use the older person's name frequently
- combine the use of written and verbal communication to increase understanding
- encourage and praise efforts to communicate.

In general, good communication is very much like good manners. If you pay attention to the other person's comfort and dignity, knowing what to do in a particular situation comes naturally.

Hearing

Many hearing problems are part of growing older. Hearing loss in older persons most often is due to aging of the hearing nerves in the inner ear. While there is no medical treatment for this type of hearing loss, other common causes of hearing loss may include a build-up of wax in the ear canal, ear infections, damage to the ear drums, a disease of the small bones in the middle ear, or problems with a hearing aid. Any loss of hearing should be evaluated by a physician. Hearing aids may be helpful in some cases, but not all hearing problems can be corrected with a hearing aid. If possible, purchase aids on a trial basis so that the correct choice of device—or no device at all—can be made. It is possible that an amplifier for the telephone or television will be more effective than a hearing aid.

Even a relatively mild hearing loss is important, since failing to hear can result in confusion and unnecessary misunderstanding. A hard-of-hearing person may feel cut off from others and feel a sense of isolation and of being alone. Depression and paranoid reactions may be related to hearing loss.

Hearing is a way to get signals from the environment and, therefore, relates to safety. It can also be embarrassing for an older person to ask people to repeat what they have said. Some hearing-impaired older persons may stop being part of the group and choose to stay alone.

It is essential that you recognize a hearing loss. The hearing-impaired person may:

- complain of occasional dizziness or ringing or buzzing or other sounds in the ears
- complain that the ears feel full or have pressure in them
- have difficulty hearing on the telephone
- have a history of noise exposure from factory or farm machinery
- lose interest in television or social activities and tend to remain alone
- have uncharacteristically loud or distorted speech
- exhibit "selective hearing," which may indicate a loss in the range of sounds they are able to hear.

Caregivers must help older persons compensate for hearing loss. When speaking, face the person directly and position yourself on the same physical level; if the person uses glasses, be sure that he or she has them on. Make sure that your mouth and lips are clearly seen to help those who lip-read, and check for glare or shadows. Arrange the environment so that the speaker's face and body can be easily seen.

It is also important to look cheerful. Your face and body expressions can enhance your communications skills. Encourage the use of nonverbal communication, such as big smiles and waving. Nonverbal communication includes body movements, facial expression, voice pitch, and sign language.

When communicating with the care recipient, ask him or her to turn off the radio or television, as background noise makes it more difficult for the hard-of-hearing person to understand conversation. Speak in a normal fashion and do not shout; shouting raises the pitch of one's voice and high frequency sounds are the most difficult for the hearing-impaired elderly to hear. If the person does not understand, rephrase what you said. Use gestures or pictures to help clarify your meaning.

Avoid chewing, eating, or covering your mouth with your hands when speaking. Stand three to six feet away from the person when speaking and avoid speaking directly into the person's ear, since that may make you harder to understand and has the potential to injure the ear further. Give the care recipient enough time to respond after you have spoken.

Make sure that the care recipient's hearing is checked regularly by his or her doctor or a hearing specialist. Place yourself near the person's hearing-aided side if a hearing aid is worn. Encourage the care recipient to wear his or her hearing aid and be sure that it has been correctly adjusted or repaired. Family members can attend rehabilitation classes for the new hearing aid user. Write down what you are saying if that will help the person understand you. In extreme cases, a pad and pencil may be the best means of communication.

Whenever possible, give the hearing-impaired person prompts about the topic of conversation. Do not change the subject abruptly. The higher-pitched voices of women and children may be harder for the hearing-impaired person to hear. Speak in a low- pitched voice, distinctly and a little more slowly than normal.

Hard-of-hearing persons may be fearful in the dark; arrange for a night light or flashlight so they will not feel isolated and alone. Emphasize activities that are visual, such as museums, books, or dance recitals. At home, door bells and telephone bells can be replaced by blinking lights.

Above all else, never talk to others about the care recipient as if he or she is not in the room.

Vision

Some normal changes occur as a person ages. These can vary widely in each individual and will require compensation that recognizes and addresses individual variations. The degree of compensation will depend on the severity of the vision loss. Older persons should have regular examinations by an ophthalmologist.

The older person who suffers from loss of vision may:

- request a brighter light for reading or handwork, or limit those activities because they are unable to see fine detail
- hold his or her book or handwork closer and closer
- find that glare on reflective surfaces causes discomfort
- stop watching television
- miss what is happening on either side but be able to see well directly ahead

- be unable to discriminate color differences
- fumble for small objects
- bump into furniture
- have difficultly seeing at night.

Caregivers can assist care recipients with vision loss by simply including them in conversations. Increase other sensory stimulation by including talking books or audio tapes as part of the daily routine.

For those with severe visual impairment, daily routine can substitute for changes usually signalled by sunup and sundown. Use clocks with black numbers on white backgrounds and telephones with large numbers. Clearly label rooms and objects and do not rearrange rooms without letting the person know what changes have been made. Rearrange rooms so that sunlight provides illumination but does not cause glare. Do not rush a visually impaired person as he or she walks, and accent step edges and head-level obstructions in the home with contrasting paint.

Identify yourself before beginning a conversation. Alert the person before touching them. A light touch on the shoulder or hand may aid a person in determining your location.

Be willing to help if necessary but do not assume that the person is unable to do things on his or her own. Be sure that clothing has pockets so important items can be near at hand and the person will not have to hunt for them.

Inability to identify colors may be a sign of vision loss rather than a sign of confusion. Pill color may not be helpful in taking the correct medication; medications should be clearly labeled.

Contrasting colors are easier to see and can be helpful in many situations, including dining, when food, plates, and utensils will be more readily visible if there is contrast among the items. Allow time for the older person to adjust to changes in light level and provide adequate natural or artificial lighting. Avoid clutter and be sure that hallways, stairs, doors, and walkways are free of obstacles.

To improve communication, sit near the person, make sure there is adequate light on your face, do not chew gum or cover your mouth, and speak at a normal rate and volume; do not shout. Remove background noises and other distractions and use verbal prompts to help the person understand the conversation.

If the person wears glasses make sure that he or she is wearing them on a regular basis. Make magnifying glasses and other vision aids readily available. If the person needs a hearing aid be sure that he or she is wearing it and that it is properly adjusted.

Taste and Smell

Sensitivity to taste and smell diminishes in the older individual as the number of taste buds and the flow of saliva decreases. Further, certain chronic conditions, such as heart disease, may require a decrease in the use of salt or other foods the person usually eats. Familiar food may become off-limits or less appetizing.

The care recipient may lose interest in eating or may forget to eat. He or she may use much more salt or other seasoning than is required to flavor food. Caregivers should check the adequacy of food available to the older person to be sure that it is sufficiently varied, well prepared and well served. Emphasis should be placed on other aspects of mealtime, such as conversation and companionship.

Check for changes in medical condition that may be signalled by a change in eating habits. Be sure that the care recipient is receiving adequate oral hygiene and dental care. If possible, plan occasional meals away from home to help sustain interest in eating.

Confusion or Reduced Intellectual Function

Many factors contribute to confusion or reduced intellectual function in the older person. While the cause may be attributed to the normal aging process in some cases, it is important to be sure that the person is checked by a physician and that medications, overall health, nutrition, mental health, substance abuse, and other factors are considered so that appropriate treatment can be provided.

Strokes are one cause of confusion in older people. They result from a disruption of blood supply to the brain and may cause temporary or permanent damage, with symptoms including paralysis or speech and vision problems. The type of disability depends on which part of the brain is affected by the stroke.

Alzheimer's disease can also be the cause of changes in a person's ability to think, remember, and interact.

The older person may:

- become forgetful
- speak without making sense
- have difficulty paying attention
- wander off or become disoriented, even in familiar surroundings
- cry or laugh at inappropriate times
- fail to understand conversation
- change his or her usual way of behaving.

To minimize confusion and encourage attempts at communication, you should attempt, whenever possible, to communicate with the care recipient in a quiet place free of noise or distraction. Be patient, always giving him or her enough time to understand and speak.

Use environmental prompts to help maintain orientation. Clocks with large, bold black numerals and hands and large calendars are helpful tools. Label drawers, cabinets, and rooms. Hang clothes according to color and consider limiting the number of choices. Label faucets and stove dials.

Call the care recipient by his or her name and remind him or her of your name often. Remind the person of the correct day, date, and year. Be consistent and try to maintain a routine that will help orient the person. When it is necessary to correct the care recipient, do so in a calm, matter-of-fact way.

Be supportive and understanding without indulging in unrealistic optimism. Before you begin speaking, identify yourself and your reason for being there. Make sure that you have the person's attention through the use of eye contact and touch. Facial expression can aid understanding.

Do not assume that the care recipient understands everything. Ask if he or she understands, be specific about what is needed from the person, and be prepared to repeat requests for information. Communicate in a calm, structured way in short, simple sentences that progress logically.

Request information. Do not order the person to answer you. Do not overreact to the use of profanity. Swearing may be normal for an older person who has difficulty monitoring and choosing words. Be sure that written material can be seen; some stroke victims can see the central portion but not see the right or left side of written material.

Give the person hints on how to say a word if you know what he or she wants to say. Just because a person can say a word one day does not mean that he or she is able to say it any time they want. If the person has little or no intelligible speech, ask questions that require a simple "yes" or "no" response. Just because a person cannot talk does not mean that he or she cannot understand. Never talk about the care recipient as if he or she was not there.

If the care recipient begins to physically wander away, seek immediate assistance from your family physician or the local Alzheimer's resource center. Only in rare instances is physical restraint appropriate.

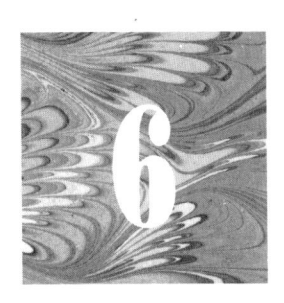

Medication Management and the Normal Aging Process

Robert J. Kassan, M.D.

There are many factors unique to the understanding of medication in the aging individual. Because of the presence of many conflicting conditions, it is important that health professionals individualize each situation in approaching the prescribing of medications.

In this age of medical specialization, it is not unusual for patients to be seen by more than one physician and to be given prescription medications by each of them. In many instances, incompatibilities between the medications can lead to a decline in the older person's health. Caregivers can play an important role in eliminating the possibility of the interference of one drug regimen with another.

It is not unusual for illnesses such as hypertension, arthritis, and diabetes to appear repeatedly from one generation to the next. Knowledge of family health history on the part of the caregiver can encourage the timely use of preventative measures that can delay the onset or lessen the impact of these conditions. If a care recipient has a family history of arthritis, encourage exercise. For diabetes and lipid disorders, encourage an appropriate diet. Persons with a family history of hypertension should restrict their salt intake.

Caregivers can also be of great assistance to care recipients by seeing that medications are used as prescribed. Medications do no good if they are left in the medicine cabinet; they can do great harm if they are used improperly. It is important that care recipients have an understanding of the purpose and action of medications. Many older persons will demand that they be given an antibiotic when they become ill. They do not understand that antibiotics are of no benefit when infections are viral in nature. They also do not understand that the long-term use of antibiotics is problematic. Caregivers can again play a key role in helping care recipients reach their therapeutic goals.

It has been shown by statistical studies that more than one-half of all patients take prescription medications incorrectly. In addition, 12 to 20 percent of patients take medications that have been prescribed for other people. Twenty-three percent of nursing home admissions are related to improper self-administration of medicines. The National Council on Patient Information and Education found that the five most common reasons for nonuse or misuse of prescribed medications are: not having prescriptions filled; taking an incorrect dose; taking the medicine at the wrong times; forgetting to take one or more doses; and stopping the medicine too soon.

Some patients intentionally decide to change the dosage or stop taking their medicine without first consulting their physician. Others save unused medicines, such as antibiotics, and self-medicate at a later date. There are at least two dangers in this practice: self-diagnosis is very seldom correct, and even in those rare instances in which it is correct, the effectiveness or therapeutic value of the medication may have expired. Expiration dates of prescription medications should be carefully monitored. If you are uncertain about the continued usefulness of a prescription, check with the pharmacist who filled it.

It is a fairly common practice among unsupervised older persons to take a "holiday" from their drug therapy. This break in the drug therapy can trigger severe adverse reactions. Typically, the "holiday" ends with the abrupt resumption of the original dosage. This is particularly dangerous with some heart medications, as sudden increases in the dosage may overstimulate the heart. For one reason or another, about one in ten patients takes too high a dose of his or her medication and flirts with the possibility of toxic reaction. Older persons who share their own or others' medications run a similar risk. There is no standard dosage for most medications. Rather, the amount prescribed is based on the age, weight, and condition of the individual to whom they are administered. Care recipients—and, for that matter, all persons—should be strongly cautioned against using prescription medications not specifically prescribed for them.

Environmental factors, too, play a role in drug interactions. The nutritional status of older persons often is precarious due to difficulties in obtaining and preparing food, limited income, loneliness, depression, or ignorance of proper nutrition. A person's diet has been shown to play an important role in determining how he or she will respond to medication. Protein deficiencies and malnutrition impair the effectiveness of drugs. Smoking has been found to have a similar effect.

Watch closely for signs of alcohol dependency. Many older persons have well-disguised drinking problems. Anyone of any age who suffers from alcohol dependency runs a tremendous health risk. But the combination of age, multiple diagnoses, and competing medications can be immediately life threatening for older persons. The use of both alcohol and tobacco is likely to be increased in the presence of loneliness and depression and can lead to complications in medication management.

Caregivers who are given the opportunity can be of great help in solving the problems of inadequate nutrition, loneliness, and depression. It is clear that the task of the caregiver does not stop with the simple administration of medications.

Enhanced quality of life is the primary goal of drug therapy in older persons. The cure of disease is often not possible, but the alleviation of symptoms can involve simple measures, often without the use of drugs. When medical therapy is required, however, caregivers and medical professionals must be vigilant in watching for the potential effects of age and disease in altering drug disposition and response.

By increasing our knowledge of the effects of drugs on older persons and by improving communication among the patient, the physician, and the caregiver, medical outcomes for older persons can be greatly improved.

Physical Changes Associated with Aging

Mrs. Garcia mentions to her daughter that she is concerned over changes in her sleeping pattern. Once a sound sleeper, she now finds that she will sleep for only four to five hours and then toss and turn restlessly until daybreak. She has noticed, too, that her appetite is not as great as it used to be and that food is losing its taste. She is most concerned, however, over the fact that she is becoming forgetful. Yesterday, she misplaced her car keys and had to reschedule an appointment at the beauty parlor. Last week, she became confused when attempting to find a Women's Club member's new home and arrived 30 minutes late. Mrs. Garcia has always prided herself on her punctuality.

Mrs. Garcia is 71 years old.

One of the great challenges to older persons' loved ones and medical care providers lies in distinguishing normal changes due to the aging process from symptoms of the onset of illness or disease. Normal biological changes, if not recognized as such, can result in the administration of unnecessary medications that may pose a hazard to an older person's health.

Is Mrs. Garcia's difficulty in sleeping due to incompatible reaction to multiple medications, or is it possible that, like many older persons, Mrs. Jones needs less sleep than she did when she was younger and more active?

Is her change in appetite a possible sign of an adverse reaction to medication with a decrease in saliva secretion resulting in dryness, or is it a result of the normal decline in the sense of smell and taste experienced by most older persons?

Is Mrs. Garcia experiencing the early signs of dementia, or is she no more forgetful than most younger persons and worrying unnecessarily? Is her difficulty in finding her friend's home due to subtle, undiagnosed changes in her eyesight?

VISION

All of us experience changes in vision as we grow older. The first thing most people notice in the way of visual change may be a diminished ability to focus on objects viewed at short range. This is called presbyopia—far-sightedness—and is due to a reduction in the ability of the eye to shift from far to near and to focus equally well at both distances.

Many older people also experience a loss in sharpness or clarity of vision at a distance. The 20/20 of "normal" vision refers to the ability to see clearly at 20 feet what should be clear at 20 feet. If one sees the chart at 20 feet, but the letters or symbols should have been seen clearly at 50 feet, a person is assigned 20/50 vision. A person whose vision, even with corrected glasses, is only 20/200 is legally blind.

At birth, we all have a transparent lens in each of our eyes but as we age, the lens begins to yellow. This yellowing begins to filter out colors at the lower end of the spectrum—violet, blue, and green. The brightness of reds, yellows, and oranges at the upper end of the spectrum are less affected and more easily discerned. Darker colors may blur together and the shapes and boundaries of similarly colored objects, shapes, or spaces may be difficult to distinguish.

Older people need more light to see well than do younger people. On average, an 80-year-old needs 200 times the wattage as a 20-year-old to see the same thing. This is due to the reduction in pupil size as a function of aging.

The two most common eye diseases in the elderly are glaucoma, an increase in pressure within the eye, and cataracts, which cause a complete shadowing of the lens. One in four persons over the age of 70 has cataracts. Glaucoma can appear in younger people as a complication of disease, such as diabetes, or as an adverse effect of a medication. But it is seen most frequently in older people. Glaucoma should be strongly suspected when there is a complaint of seeing a halo around light sources such as headlights. Untreated, it can result in blindness. Screening for glaucoma should begin between ages 30 and 35.

Both glaucoma and cataracts can be dealt with either by eyeglasses or surgery so that activities of daily living and social functioning can be restored to a relatively normal level, but:

- reading and finely detailed close work may be limited
- night driving may need to be avoided for safety's sake
- in a darkened restaurant decorated in blue and green, the older person may not see hallways, stairs, and open spaces as differentiated, while in a brightly lit supermarket, the glare and very small price labels may prove discouraging.

Caregivers and health care providers should be aware of behavior that signals a loss of acuity, color perception, or the inability to adjust vision from distant to close objects. Helping the care recipient understand and adapt to these changes may be as important as corrective glasses or a new prescription.

HEARING

Hearing impairment has a profound effect on older persons because it cuts them off from communication with others, from hearing and enjoying music and television, and even from the sounds their own bodies make.

An inability to hear what is being said can cause older persons to become suspicious and to be vigilant in trying to observe their environment. Unfortunately, the label "paranoid" is often attached to the older hearing-impaired person. Hearing only a part of what was said, or hearing it incorrectly, leads the listener to make what may seem to the speaker to be wildly inappropriate responses. More often than not, the speaker will get no response and will subsequently discontinue his or her attempts to communicate. The result is a withdrawal of the hearing impaired from social interaction.

The use of mechanical hearing aids can improve hearing, but the need remains for the speaker to speak louder, slower, and more clearly. Unfortunately, the use of hearing aids can result in an accentuation of extraneous noises.

The onset of hearing changes can begin as early as age 20 and is more common in men. Thirty percent of older persons report hearing-related disabilities by age 65.

The most common hearing impairment is presbyacusia. Persons with this condition experience difficulties with speech discrimination—high-frequency sounds are not heard so that speech is heard in a distorted fashion. Complicating the problem is another impairment, recruitment, which lowers the point at which noise becomes painfully loud to a level very close to that needed for a person to hear speech. This condition not only presents an obstacle to understanding speech, but also to the use of amplification such as hearing aids.

Tinnitus, or noise heard in the ear, is a symptom rather than a disease. It is more common in the elderly and often appears as a constant or intermittent ringing. It is often untreatable. Tinnitus can accompany deafness and is extremely stressful.

Caregivers and health care providers generally find that hearing loss is more difficult to deal with than vision loss. Deafness may be an invisible handicap, leading to withdrawal, isolation, and a lack of responsiveness on the part of the care recipient.

JOINTS, MUSCLES, AND BONES

Disorders of joints, muscles, and bones are common reasons for older persons' physician visits. They are the leading cause of the reduction in older persons' activities of daily living. About one-half of all persons aged 70 or older are affected by progressive disability syndrome, leading to weakness, motion restriction, deformity, and chronic pain.

Arthritis, rheumatism, and rheumatic disease are interchangeable terms for a number of diverse medical conditions with the common element of pain and a disabling of the joints or supportive tissues. More than 100 medical conditions fall into this category. Because each of these conditions is different, the approach to the treatment, control, and management varies. It is of paramount importance that a specific diagnosis be made and understood.

The effects of normal aging occur as a result of decreases in bulk, strength, and muscle endurance (myopathy), the thinning and shrinking of bone mass (osteopenia and osteoporosis), and loss of the fluid that lubricates joints accompanied by the hardening and splintering of cartilage covering bone endings (osteoarthritis). These changes represent more than normal wear and tear on the body. They represent disease processes that can be prevented and treated. A secondary—and potentially life-threatening—effect of these musculoskeletal changes is the increased likelihood of fractures from falling.

Prevention and treatment of musculoskeletal problems is simple: exercise. Older persons who continue a regular program of exercise will lose less bulk, strength, and endurance and slow or even reverse the shrinking and thinning of bone mass. Even the deformities of osteoarthritis and rheumatoid arthritis can be avoided by exercise.

Caregivers and health care providers should encourage older persons to exercise, to eat calcium rich foods, and to take vitamin supplements containing vitamin D. They can also help by assisting them in obtaining aids to mobility and strength, which can keep them active and alert.

THE CARDIOVASCULAR SYSTEM

Cardiovascular disease is the leading cause of death in older persons. Yet many cardiovascular conditions reflect normal changes due to aging in the heart and blood vessels.

As the heart ages, the heart wall thickens, valve functioning decreases, and the heart beats more slowly. This slowing results in a decrease in the supply of oxygenated blood to body tissues, with a subsequent loss of energy and a more rapid onset of fatigue.

Arteriosclerosis, a narrowing of the arteries by deposits of cholesterol, is made worse by the normal aging of the arterial wall, which becomes more rigid. This affects the heart by decreasing the flow of blood and oxygen to the heart muscle. This combination of reduced blood flow and narrower arteries contributes to high blood pressure, also known as hypertension. If left untreated, hypertension can lead to enlargement of the heart, kidney failure, blindness, stroke, and congestive heart failure.

Hypertension can be controlled by a reduction in salt intake, weight loss, exercise, and stress management. Medications such as diuretics (water pills), beta blockers, calcium channel blockers, and angiotensin converter enzyme (ACE) may also be prescribed. Generally, the avoidance of foods that are high in cholesterol, smoking cessation, and a reduction in alcohol intake will help control existing hypertension and prevent its onset.

A decrease in the flow of blood to the heart muscle and brain can result in pain, known as angina, and transient ischemic attacks (TIAs), which are sometimes referred to as mini-strokes. TIAs are caused by a temporary interruption in the flow of blood to the brain. Both angina and TIAs can cause permanent damage to the heart or brain, ultimately leading to heart attack or stroke. Both can be devastating, with stroke leading to paralysis, an absence or numbness of feeling in the limbs, and the inability to speak.

It is essential that caregivers seek regular medical attention for loved ones suffering from cardiovascular disease.

THE PULMONARY SYSTEM

As we age, problems arise that can cause difficulty in breathing, both at rest and during periods of exertion. Older persons have a greater tendency to develop lung infections because of more sedentary lifestyles and generally experience a decrease in resistance to infection. Expansion of the chest and the resulting introduction of fresh oxygen to replace carbon dioxide is reduced. The walls of the lungs thin and small blood vessels are destroyed.

Repeated infections of the bronchial tubes can cause a thickening of the walls, resulting in difficulty in breathing with any increase in exertion. This condition results in further thinning of the lung walls and leads to emphysema or chronic pulmonary obstructive disease. Often, medications aimed at relaxing or expanding the bronchial passages are prescribed, but their use should be evaluated according to the older person's general medical condition and the use of other medications. Older persons may also develop allergies that can be treated only through elimination of the offending substance from the surrounding atmosphere or through measures that desensitize him or her to the allergen causing the problem.

THE GASTROINTESTINAL SYSTEM

It is important to understand the changes that take place in the gastrointestinal (GI) tract in order to understand and appreciate the effect of medications in older persons. There is no question that GI tract problems are more prevalent as we age. Fewer than 5 percent of people under 45 years of age complain of GI symptoms or disorders, while 25 percent of those over age 65 have related complaints.

A great many changes occur with aging. The amount of saliva secreted in the mouth may decrease. This not only results in difficulty in chewing and swallowing food, but also reduces the availability of enzymes, which begin the digestive process. Saliva also has an antibiotic action that prevents infection and decay in the gums and teeth. Degeneration of smell and taste receptors cause a decline in taste at about age 50. By age 80, many people have difficulty in distinguishing between sweet, sour, and salty foods. This can lead to a decrease in appetite.

Older persons also complain of difficulty in swallowing, due to thickening of the esophagus wall and the growth of a skin-like lining, and an increase in food regurgitation, due to a decrease in saliva secretion. Muscle tone in the diaphragm decreases, resulting in a dislocation of the upper end of the stomach into the chest cavity. This can cause heartburn, chest pain, and belching.

With aging, peristaltic action, or normal movement of the bowel due to rhythmic muscular contraction, decreases. Frequently, this decrease is the result of lack of fiber in the diet, inactivity, or a decrease in food intake due to illness. In many instances, this results in the most common GI complaint among the elderly, constipation. Other complaints include diverticulosis, the development of pouches in the intestinal wall, and hemorrhoids, the swelling of the blood vessels in the anal area as a result of straining. A decrease in the production and secretion of hydrochloric acid, which is necessary for the digestion of protein, may also occur.

Most of the GI symptoms related to normal aging can be controlled by eating smaller amounts of food more frequently, eating slowly, and drinking more fluids; weight loss; and sleeping with the head elevated at night. Indigestion may decrease and ulcers may improve with the elimination of smoking, caffeine, alcohol, and fat, rich, or spicy foods and the use of medications that control acid, such as H-2 blockers or antacids. Changes in the upper gastrointestinal tract mean that medications in liquid form may be better tolerated and more effective in the treatment of most conditions.

THE CENTRAL NERVOUS SYSTEM

The central nervous system is made up of nerve cells (neurons) and nerve tissues in the spinal cord and brain. It undergoes progressive changes with age, most frequently evidenced by cognitive and psychological changes. Circulatory changes in the brain can cause many of these symptoms. Any means by which circulation can be improved will result in improved function, as long as no permanent damage has occurred. Many of these changes can be minimized through the use of available medications.

The disturbance of sleeping patterns is a reflection of the normal changes that occur in the brain throughout the aging process. While older persons make up about 12 percent of the population nationwide, they account for 40 percent of the consumption of sleep inducing drugs. Warm milk, which contains an amino acid, tryptophan, which is helpful in inducing sleep, may be a good substitute for some older persons. But tryptophan has recently been taken off the market because of its link to symptoms including low-grade fever, severe fatigue, and skin rash.

Caregivers should become knowledgeable about the specific condition of the person who is under their care. Regardless of the diagnosis, there is one overriding element of care to which every patient responds: the demonstration of empathy for discomfort and pain, accompanied by the wholehearted giving of emotional support.

This translates into "tender loving care."

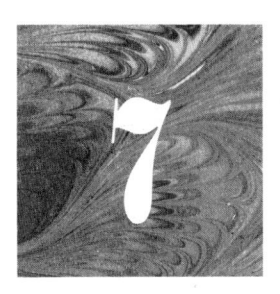

Alcohol and Substance Abuse in the Elderly

Jayne LaRue, M.S.W.

Dave began drinking beer at the age of 15. At age 72, he continues to drink, telling himself and concerned family members that he doesn't have a drinking problem. When he was younger, Dave had difficulty keeping a job and relations with his now deceased wife and children were strained. Most of his six children avoid him because of his mean temperament and abusive nature when he is drinking—which seems to be most of the time in recent months.

Last week, Dave was diagnosed with end-stage liver disease related to alcohol consumption. Dave refuses to accept the diagnosis and blames his failing health on his diet and on his youngest daughter, Mary Beth, who, he says, ignores him. When Dave left the hospital, his first stop was a liquor store, where he bought a fifth of whiskey and two six packs of beer.

When Mary Beth learned that Dave had sought medical attention, she approached him about his drinking and expressed her concern for his well-being. He responded angrily, saying that whiskey and beer are not his problem—but meddling do-gooders are.

Martha, 67, and her husband, Mitch, relocated to Florida six years ago, after Mitch's retirement. They were happy with their life in a Southwest Florida trailer park and enjoyed an active social life. But last year, Mitch suffered a stroke and Martha was unable to care for him at home. Mitch was placed in a nursing home about a 45-minute drive from their retirement community.

Mitch's stroke brought a new set of responsibilities and challenges, which were overwhelming to Martha, who had been a homemaker. First, there was managing their limited financial resources. Then there was the challenge of getting to the nursing home for daily visits. Martha did not like to drive and seldom had since the move to Florida. It was particularly difficult when her arthritis flared up and, recently, the pain had intensified. A sympathetic neighbor urged her to try a daily shot of bourbon for the pain, a remedy she had learned from her doctor when she was in her twenties.

Martha took the neighbor's advice and began a late afternoon "medicinal" regimen. She found that it not only helped her pain, but that it also made her feel better—that is, less depressed, more sociable, and less anxious. As time passed, however, she found that a single shot of bourbon didn't always have the desired effect. She began taking her bourbon earlier in the day and found that two shots, sometimes more, were more effective in controlling her arthritic pain.

Martha's anxiety increased and she had difficulty sleeping. She found herself crying frequently because she felt that the world was against her; nobody understood her situation. Martha began to forget simple chores and did not take her medications correctly. She feared that she was going crazy and, as a last resort, decided to go to her doctor. She told him of her difficulties and of her "self-medication."

Luckily, Martha's doctor recognized that her physical and psychological problems were magnified because of her alcohol use. He encouraged her to discontinue the bourbon and referred her to an alcohol counselor who could help her stop drinking and address her problems of loneliness, isolation from family, loss of her husband as partner, and depression.

Ed, 75, liked to have a drink with the boys now and then. Whenever he drank he would get drunk, but his drinking was so rare that it never disturbed his family life.

After his wife's death, however, Ed began to drink more frequently and more heavily. He no longer felt the need to control his drinking, because he felt there was nothing to worth staying sober for. This continued for several years, and Ed's physical health deteriorated rapidly.

Although his daughter came by once a week, it never occurred to her that his drinking was a problem. She felt that if it would help him get over her mother's death there was no harm in it. For a time, he was able to hide the extent to which he drank from her, but he eventually became confused and incontinent.

At that point his daughter realized he had a problem, and because of his rapidly deteriorating condition, she no longer thought he could care for himself at home. With great regret, she made the decision to place her father in a nursing home.

Alcoholism and substance abuse are not exclusively problems of the young. Unfortunately, however, all too often symptoms of abuse are overlooked or misdiagnosed in the elderly—sometimes with tragic consequences.

Perhaps you have been experiencing difficulty managing the person you are caring for and are not sure why. Or, perhaps you know that your loved one has a problem with drugs or alcohol but don't know where to turn for help. This chapter is designed as a resource for you: to define alcohol and substance abuse or misuse and to give you an idea of where to turn for assistance.

Alcoholism

There are two types of drinking: social and problem. When drunk in small, controlled amounts, alcohol can have many pleasant effects, including enhancing one's ability to relax, communicate, and feel comfort with the environment.

Alcohol intake becomes a problem when it is consumed consistently, over a long period of time, without control, resulting in life problems and patterns of behavior that become a serious threat to the drinker's physical and mental health. What began as a means to "feel better" can spiral into a vicious cycle of drinking to "feel normal." Usually, the result is "feeling worse."

Unfortunately, the process can be slow and evasive. The alcoholic may not believe that he or she has a problem, even if friends and family are fully aware and confront him or her with their concern.

Alcoholism among the elderly is conservatively estimated to affect 2 to 10 percent of the general population and is higher among widowers, those with physical problems, and those with criminal histories. It is estimated to be as high as 40% among those elderly who are institutionalized.

Alcoholics are at great risk of becoming injured, ill, or in need of institutionalization due to physical and mental deterioration. While alcohol use usually is discontinued in an institutional setting, the ramifications of use still evidence themselves.

There is no absolute definition of alcoholism in that it cannot be quantified by a set number of drinks. In fact, it varies for each individual. Generally, the indication that someone has a drinking problem is that he or she develops major life problems that are directly related to the use of alcohol. Examples include: divorce or marital separation, compromised physical or mental health; loss of job; and driving while intoxicated, which results in problems with the law.

It should be noted, however, that some of the indicators that apply in younger people, such as, loss of job, family, and friends may not apply to the elderly because they can be considered normal consequences of aging. In fact, these events may precipitate problem drinking in some elderly individuals.

Indicators of alcohol abuse in the elderly include:

- health problems, both mental and physical
- financial difficulties
- loss of ties to family and friends due to their inability to cope with the behaviors directly related to the drinking
- the smell of alcohol
- frequent intoxication
- shakes and tremors when unable to drink
- frequent falls, bruises, burns, and home accidents
- rapid changes in mood
- inability to control bowel and bladder function.

One of these symptoms, alone, does not necessarily indicate a drinking problem. A problem may exist if several are occurring together and a pattern of behavior is emerging.

It is important to identify the elderly drinker, since there can be many adverse physical and psychological consequences due to alcohol abuse. Physically, alcohol can mask disease processes including, brain, liver, and kidney damage, exacerbating these conditions or creating new problems.

The pain that accompanies an angina attack could go unnoticed due to alcohol's diminishing of one's awareness of pain. Furthermore, alcohol abuse can cause the misdiagnosis of medical problems. Common characteristics of organic brain syndrome such as impairment of memory, orientation, intellectual functioning, and judgment also are characteristic of the dementia associated with alcohol overuse. These conditions require different courses of treatment.

Malnutrition also is a concern in the elderly alcoholic. Some alcoholics intentionally will not eat in an effort to increase the effects of the alcohol. Others may experience a decrease in appetites that may result in their not eating an adequate, well-balanced diet. Because of this they are not receiving the proper nutrition. Coupled with the effects of alcoholism, a poor diet can cause a myriad of physical and mental problems for the elderly person.

Alcohol also impairs judgment, increasing the risk of falls and traffic accidents. Both can lead to injury of the alcoholic or others.

If the physical consequences aren't enough, the psychological can often be overwhelming. It is the psychological aspects that can lead the individual into the dangerous cycle of drinking to "feel better."

Depression is a major problem for many elderly people, particularly for late onset drinkers, who drink in response to their depression because they are not dealing with their losses related to aging. Because alcohol is a depressant it actually *increases* depression, it does not alleviate it.

Alcoholism can cause insomnia and a general loss of interest in life. It also can promote undesirable personality traits that may cause tension and difficulty with friends and family. Combined, these may cause the alcoholic to become withdrawn and isolated from the rest of the world.

The final and, perhaps, most frightening consequence of untreated alcoholism is suicide. Elderly males commit suicide more than any other sub-group. Using alcohol as a means to cope with problems only increases psychological despair and frustration. Suicide, therefore, is a very real concern for elderly alcoholics.

Drinkers generally fall into one of three categories:

EARLY ONSET

Early onset alcoholics, like Dave, have a long history of drinking, which began at an early age. They have continued to drink regardless of the problems it has created. They have somehow survived into old age and continue to drink regardless of the consequences, just as they did in their younger years.

This type of alcoholic is the least likely to seek treatment and are very difficult for the caregiver to manage because of their shared history and unresolved conflict. Additionally, early onset drinkers will strongly deny that they have a drinking problem until a medical crisis arises. Sometimes, they will continue to use alcohol even against medical advice.

If left untreated, early onset alcoholics either die or end up in institutional settings. Once in treatment, however, they can quit drinking and make significant life improvements.

LATE ONSET

Late onset drinkers begin to drink later in life in an effort to cope with age-related losses and stress. Alcohol is their means of escape from their problems. Often, like Martha, the late onset drinker is reacting to the loss of a spouse, child, friend, neighborhood or support system. The pain of these losses is very real and can be paralyzing.

Fortunately, late onset drinkers are the most amenable to treatment, with alcohol use a symptom of the underlying problems. Once those problems are addressed or alleviated, it is likely they will no longer feel the need to drink.

INTERMITTENT DRINKER

Intermittent drinkers, like Ed, have had periods in their lives during which they drank heavily, generally when there has been some life difficulty or crisis. The periods of problem drinking are combined with periods of sobriety.

As older persons experience losses, they may have increased difficulty coping and "turn to the bottle" for comfort and as a means of escape. Usually they are less successful in controlling their drinking because many of the "control factors"—such as job, family, friends, and mobility—are now gone. Had Ed's problem with alcohol been identified earlier he may not have needed nursing home placement. His underlying reason for drinking was the unresolved grief he had in connection with his wife's death.

Where to Turn for Assistance

Although it may be difficult to get older alcoholics into treatment, once involved, they are more likely to complete their course of therapy than any other group. Late onset drinkers are the easiest to encourage to seek treatment as the pattern of drinking is not long-standing.

There are a number of options for treatment:

ALCOHOLICS ANONYMOUS (AA)

This is a valuable resource, and groups often meet at community senior centers. This is a particularly good option for the mobile elderly because it provides peer support and counseling.

By interacting with other elderly alcoholics, individuals increase their contact with the outside world and become less isolated. But attendance can not be forced. The individual must admit that he or she has a drinking problem.

AL ANON

This group is designed to provide assistance and support to those who are affected by the alcoholism of a friend or family member. The alcoholic does not have to be in treatment in order for the caregiver to attend meetings.

Al Anon meetings provide information, peer support, and advice. Members may be able to help caregivers see whether and how they are enabling the alcoholic to continue drinking, as well as, what they can do to improve their quality of life.

COUNSELING

Counseling has many different forms: individual, group, couples, and family. Depending on the issues that the alcoholic and the caregiver need to work on will determine the type of counseling that will be most effective. When looking for a counselor it is important to find someone who is knowledgeable about the unique issues associated with aging as well as alcohol and substance abuse. Sometimes these services can be provided in the home.

SUPPORTIVE SERVICES

Case management services can provide assistance with meals, housing, cleaning, transportation and other needs of the elderly. Often, the provision of these services can increase an older person's functioning and independence, alleviating some of the daily stress in their lives.

INPATIENT TREATMENT

Inpatient treatment ranges from three to 28 days and usually involves a period of "drying out." During this phase, which involves complete abstinence from alcohol, some alcoholics experience withdrawal symptoms. The most common symptom is delirium tremors (DTs).

While in inpatient treatment, patients will be monitored and given the appropriate medication to minimize the effects of alcohol withdrawal. Patients will be involved in individual and group counseling, and also may participate in AA meetings.

OUTPATIENT TREATMENT

Outpatient treatment also involves complete abstinence from alcohol, with medications used in controlling withdrawal symptoms administered on an outpatient basis.

Patients must come to the outpatient facility on a daily basis, usually for the entire day. There, they receive individual and group counseling and are monitored for physical difficulties. Some programs encourage AA participation in the evenings, while others may hold AA meetings during the day.

Substance Abuse

Alcohol use in the elderly generally does not occur without the use of other drugs, either prescribed or over-the-counter (OTC). Although some elderly people abuse illicit drugs (i.e., marijuana, LSD, cocaine, or heroin), this is usually a carry-over from their youth and they generally have been or continue to be in trouble with the law.

Although the elderly comprise 11 percent of the general population they account for 25 percent of all prescription and over the counter drug purchases. Because of this, the potential for misuse or abuse is great. Abuse occurs when an individual intentionally uses drugs incorrectly in order to achieve a desired effect. Misuse denotes using drugs incorrectly without the intent to knowingly abuse them.

Examples of misuse and abuse include:

- John, an aging criminal, who routinely purchases marijuana and cocaine for personal use
- Ralph, who falsifies his prescriptions in order to obtain a higher dosage of his anxiety medication
- Alice, who goes to several doctors with the same complaint in order to receive multiple prescriptions of the same medication
- Beverly, whose friend loaned her an old prescription of muscle relaxants for the pain she was having in her back

- Hazel, who takes half of the prescribed dosage of her medications in order to save on prescription bills
- Beatrice, who washes down her anti-anxiety medication with a glass of white wine
- Joe, 65 years old, who smokes two packs of cigarettes and consumes a bottle of cough syrup daily to control his cough. Although the package labeling says to see a doctor if the symptoms are not alleviated within seven days, Joe has done this for the past three months. He has found that he craves the cough syrup, although he realizes it does nothing for his emphysema. It's no wonder: the cough syrup contains 25 percent alcohol.

Although some of these scenarios may seem harmless, the consequences can be detrimental for the user. Just as with alcohol, drugs are absorbed and excreted differently by the elderly than they are by young adults. Therefore, using drugs other than as prescribed can cause both physical and psychological problems, regardless of whether the individual intended to misuse them.

The most common misuse of drugs in the elderly is under-use—not taking the full amount of a prescription in an effort to make it last or because of undesirable side effects. This can be detrimental to the user, in that the drug therapy will be ineffective and may cause a life-threatening situation.

Sometimes misuse can lead to abuse, as in the case of Joe. Had he followed the directions on the label, Joe would have seen a doctor after seven days and would have avoided addiction to the alcohol contained in the cough syrup. Frequently, there is a fine line between abuse and misuse.

Drugs also can be misused due to physician error or to a physician's lack of knowledge about all of the medications an individual is taking. To avoid this, inform all physicians involved in the care of your older loved one of all medications being taken. When in doubt, ask your pharmacist to check the list of medications to make sure none of the drugs taken in combination will have adverse affects. Finally, if any physical or cognitive changes are noticed, *contact the prescribing physician immediately.*

Because the elderly use large quantities of over-the-counter and prescription drugs, they are at a high risk of drug interactions. These may go unnoticed because the symptoms are similar to those rightly or wrongly associated with old age—forgetfulness, weakness, anxiety, insomnia, and anorexia. It is imperative that drugs be taken as prescribed under the supervision of a physician who is aware of all medications that are being taken.

Where to turn for assistance

The course of treatment or assistance will depend in large part on whether your loved one is abusing or misusing drugs. If he or she is abusing drugs, then the addiction and the reasons for the abuse must be addressed. If the person is misusing their drugs, certain guidelines and behavior modifications could curtail the problem.

NARCOTICS ANONYMOUS (NA)
Narcotics Anonymous is a resource similar to AA in which people who are addicted to narcotic drugs gather to counsel and support one another in an effort to refrain from using. Before attending a session, check to find out the age range of participants. It may not be suitable for elderly persons.

THE PHYSICIAN
The physician is a valuable resource in this matter because she can advise the patient as to how to correctly take their drugs, as well as monitor their usage and the effects.

THE PHARMACIST
The pharmacist also can help the patient monitor the adverse effects a combination of drugs may have and provide information on how to more effectively administer medication.

THE NATIONAL CLEARINGHOUSE FOR DRUG ABUSE INFORMATION
The Clearinghouse has a free booklet titled *Elder-Ed* that is designed to help older persons manage their medicines more effectively. It is easy to read and provides simple suggestions. The booklet may be obtained by writing: NCDAI, Post Office Box 416, Kensington, MD, 20795.

OTHER RESOURCES
As with alcoholism, other resources include counseling, supportive services, and inpatient and outpatient treatment.

Taking Care of the Caregiver

Caregivers always try to make everything better. This may not be possible when their loved one suffers from alcohol or substance addiction.

While it may be possible to attempt to limit the availability of alcohol or other drugs, it is important to realize that alcoholism and substance abuse is as much a symptom as it is a problem. Caregivers may serve their loved ones best by seeking help for themselves through counseling and/or by attending Al Anon meetings.

If your loved one will not agree to seek help, and if you determine that he or she is at risk to himself or others, it may be necessary to seek outside assistance from the court system.

It is important to monitor the care recipient for symptoms of alcohol and drug abuse or misuse. However, it also is important to monitor yourself for the same symptoms. Caregiving can be an exhausting and, often times, overwhelming experience. If you believe that you may be in need of assistance, then seek out help. Maintaining your own physical and mental well-being is as important as caring for your loved one.

References

Amodeo, M. (1990). "Treating the Late Life Alcoholic: Guidelines for Working Through Denial and Integrating Individual, Family and Group Approaches." *Journal of Geriatric Psychiatry*, 23, 91–105.

Gerbino, P. (1982). "Complications of Alcohol Use Combined With Drug Therapy in the Elderly." *Journal of the American Geriatrics Society*, 30, 88–93.

Lawson, G. & Lawson A. *Alcoholism and Substance Abuse in Special Populations.* Rockville, MD: Aspen Publishers (1989).

Mayer, M. (1979). "Alcohol and the Elderly: A Review." *Health and Social Work*, 4, 128–141.

National Institute on Aging. *Self Care and Self Help Groups For the Elderly: A Directory.* Washington, D.C. (1985).

National Institute on Alcohol and Alcoholism. (1988). "Alcohol and Aging." *Alcohol Alert*, 2, 1–4.

National Institute on Alcohol and Alcoholism. (1989). "Alcohol and Cognition." *Alcohol Alert*, 4, 1–4.

Newman-Aspel, M. (1990). "Two Cases of Late Life Alcoholism." *Journal of Geriatric Psychiatry*, 23, 107–116.

Pruzinsky, E. (1987). "Alcohol and the Elderly: An Overview of Problems in the Elderly and Implications for Social Work Practice." *Journal of Gerontological Social Work*, 11, 81–93.

Schuckit, M. (1977). "Geriatric Alcoholism and Drug Abuse." *The Gerontologist*, 17, 168–174.

Sumberg, D. (1985). "Social Work With Elderly Alcoholics: Some Practical Considerations." *Gerontological Social Work Practice in the Community*, 169–180.

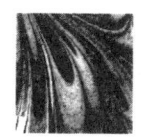

Profile

"Bill" and "Wilma" were married while still in their teens. Both are now aged 75. Wilma has lived in a nursing home since age 67. Bill stays busy in a self-employed capacity as a marketing consultant. Although he retired a few years ago from full-time employment, he explains that he must continue his self-employment in order to pay for Wilma's care and medical expenses.

Wilma was diagnosed with Alzheimer's disease while in her early sixties. The first symptom was failing memory. Soon she no longer remembered how to get a drink of water at the kitchen sink or how to drive to familiar destinations. Other changes took place at a rapid pace until it became unsafe for her to be alone at home, where she fell on the steps or often hurt herself in the kitchen.

"The biggest hurt for me is the loneliness, not having anybody to share with," says Bill. "We were so close. I can hardly remember not being married." For a number of years they ran a business together in addition to his full-time job. "She was so smart, so active and capable." Now she is unable to communicate, recognizes no one and requires 24-hour care.

Bill managed to take care of Wilma at home for two-and one-half years. He considered having three shifts a day with her, but the cost was prohibitive. At age 67, she entered an adult congregate living facility (ACLF). This did not work out, however, as the skilled care that Wilma soon needed was not available. She fell and broke her hip and had to move to a nursing home.

Keeping Wilma in the nursing

home has been extraordinarily difficult for Bill. For a while, Wilma would become upset and agitated when he visited; after a while, the nurse suggested to Bill that it would be better for her if he did not visit so often. He is heartbroken over her rapidly deteriorating condition.

"She can't walk or talk. Her skin is now paper thin and tears easily," he says, choking back tears. "The main thing is making her as comfortable as possible."

Bill used to go to a support group. It was helpful to share with other people going through the same thing. One man in the group, he recalls, "made a career of it and died."

Bill's and Wilma's children are scattered geographically. One granddaughter lives near enough to visit on occasion. Bill would like to try to find happiness in a new relationship. But few women his age are willing to risk a long-term relationship with a married man, even when they know his situation.

Bill faces the necessity of having to continue working even though he is 75. He hopes that he will be able to continue to earn enough to support himself and Wilma's care. He worries constantly about expenses. The nursing home costs $2,400 a month. With medicines, physicians' fees, emergency costs, and extras, Wilma's care costs about $30,000 a year.

Bill feels strongly about the unfairness of government policy. He has received "not one nickel" from Medicare, and he is angered by the fact that "seven times as much money is spent every year on AIDS research as is spent on Alzheimer's research."

From his experience, Bill offers this advice:

Never promise not to put a loved one in a nursing home. "You may need to sooner than you think."

"You just can't let yourself brood over it. Your life goes on."

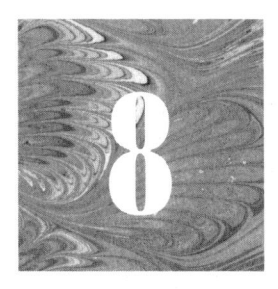

# Dementia and the Caregiver

George F. Slade, M.D.

Between 1940 and 1980, there was an eight-fold increase in the number of people over age 65. Regrettably, the number of persons with dementia increased proportionately.

Dementia is a clinical term used to describe a usually progressive mental deterioration, including loss of memory and loss of cognitive function and the resulting inability to carry out the activities of daily living.

Dementia is not one illness. Rather, it comes in many forms caused both by disease and, in some cases, medication. A recent survey of dementia showed that drugs may be the root cause of one in ten dementia cases. It is generally held, however, that a number of contributing factors combine to cause the onset of dementia. The two most common forms of dementia are senile dementia of the Alzheimer's type (SDAT) and vascular or multi-infarct dementia (MID).

The demented brain is the equivalent of a rusted television antenna precariously perched on the roof of a house. Television reception is poor when there are strong winds, rain, snow, excessive heat, or other environmental factors. In persons with dementia, both the antenna and television are housed in the brain. The ravages of nature that can affect television reception are replaced in the brain by a fear of darkness, unfamiliar places, or strangers. New locations or subtle changes in the lighting or color of rooms trigger anxiety, fear, and pain. The demented person's "reception" may be so poor that he or she becomes disoriented and confused. As the disease progresses, the demented person becomes less able to control certain basic emotions and begins to misinterpret many sensory stimuli.

About 5 percent of Americans aged 65 suffer from some form of dementia. That number increases to 20 percent by age 85. In some dementia subtypes, such as familial Alzheimer's disease, the incidence of dementia at age 85 in immediate family members may reach 50 percent. SDAT accounts for 50 to 60 percent of all cases of dementia that have been confirmed at autopsy; MID accounts for about 18 percent. To complicate matters, the two may occur together.

Even though Alzheimer's disease is the largest single cause of dementia in developed countries, there is still only a limited understanding of its cause. Even experienced neurologists can have difficulty making the correct diagnosis, given the large number of conditions that cause dementia. There is no treatment to alleviate the major symptoms of the disease, but current research is likely to change this gloomy picture and bring a fuller understanding of Alzheimer's disease.

SDAT is an age-related disease, but it is not an inevitable consequence of aging. Consider for a moment the health status of Bob Hope, George Burns, Pablo Picasso, Pablo Casals, and Eubie Blake in their later years. Theirs represents a more normal aging process. Clearly, SDAT is distinct from normal aging of the brain.

Intellectual decline in SDAT is correlated with the extent of pathologic changes in the brain: the more significant the changes, the more devastating the dementia. Genetic and unknown environmental factors predispose some people to the disease, but there is no convincing evidence that psychosocial factors increase the likelihood of the occurrence of dementia. It is a major public health problem. More than 500,000 Americans are believed to be severely afflicted with the disease.

SDAT accounts for 40 to 50 percent of nursing home admissions and more than 100,000 excess deaths per year. The number of SDAT cases will triple by the year 2050 if prevention or effective treatment are not discovered.

Anyone with older relatives or friends knows that the aging process involves a normal slowing of intellectual processes and a degree of mild forgetfulness. Generally, this falls under the heading "benign senescent forgetfulness," characterized by the inability to find the correct word, to remember the name of an acquaintance, or to recollect details of a recent event. In and of itself, this is not indicative of progressive deterioration and is a normal part of aging. Still, our knowledge of the impact of normal aging on neurological function is slim.

In the few long-term, cross-sectional studies that have been performed evaluating functions that decline with age, it is apparent that vocabulary, information, comprehension, and memory for digits show little or no change between ages 25 and 75. Yet the speed of handwriting, digit symbol substitution, and small coordinated movements of the extremities may show as much as a 20 to 40 percent decline during these years.

The differentiation between the onset of dementia and simple forgetfulness involves an assessment of the severity of the memory disorder and the degree to which this impairment interferes with functioning. The presence and severity of other cognitive dysfunctions is also considered. Frequently, early impairment of financial management abilities is noted in connection with dementias. It is not generally present in normal aging. This change may be followed by an inability to select appropriate clothes and difficulties with other daily living decision-making.

Disorders of language also play an important part in dementia, affecting the order of language, whether it is written, spoken, read, or heard. A demented person with aphasia may be unable to understand words or sentences. Similarly, reading may not be understood and writing may be disturbed. In some forms of dementia, all aspects of language may be affected. Other manifestations of dementia include the inability to plan, predict, and intellectualize.

Too often, we tend to equate intelligence with memory, when in reality all aspects of cognitive dysfunction may be affected as dementia evolves. While memory dysfunction may be seen as an isolated phenomenon early in the disease, it is not necessarily indicative of dementia or dementing illness.

In the general population, the genetic risk for Alzheimer's disease is 10 to 15 percent. For some families, the risk that siblings or children will develop the disease after age 85 is as high as 50 percent; in other families, there is virtually no risk. Most close family members of Alzheimer's patients will not develop the disease, but recent studies suggest a twofold risk over the general population.

There is a strong association between Down's Syndrome, a genetic chromosomal abnormality, and Alzheimer's disease. The frequency of Alzheimer's dementia is increased dramatically in patients with Down's Syndrome, particularly in those over age 40. Researchers have also reported a similar fingerprint pattern in Alzheimer's and Down's Syndrome patients, which suggests that there may be a genetic linkage between the two.

Stages of Dementia

Progressive dementias are classified into several stages. Understanding these stages can prepare caregivers for the changes in behavior and self-care ability that occur as the disease progresses. It is important to note that not everyone suffering from dementia experiences these symptoms.

STAGE I

The onset of dementia is insidious. Its symptoms are subtle and deceptive. Frequently, friends, family members, and even the patient may be unaware that a problem exists or may be unable to pinpoint the problem if they suspect one. Symptoms in Stage I include loss of recent memory, which may at first be nothing more than a nuisance, and mild language disturbances, such as difficulty in sequencing speech or words. A previously articulate person may choose a word that is inappropriate in the context in which it is used or may mispronounce a word. Absentmindedness also becomes apparent.

In Stage I, the ability to concentrate decreases and there may be mild disorientation as to time and location. The way one acts and dresses may reflect carelessness and he or she may appear to be slower in learning and in reacting to environmental changes. At this stage, the dementia victim will prefer the familiar and shun anything that is unfamiliar. In fact, unfamiliar activity may make him or her extremely anxious and cause withdrawal from friends and family members.

Decision-making tends to become more difficult in this stage. Paranoia and delusions of persecution may come and go. Errors in judgment and calculation may cause the person to give up his or her own financial bookkeeping. Most frequently, there are changes resulting in frustration, depression, or inappropriate anger.

One of the most difficult aspects of the onset of dementia is the exaggeration of the affected person's worst personality characteristics. If the caregiver has had problems with aspects of the care recipient's personality prior to the onset of dementia, it is almost certain that these problems will be exacerbated.

STAGE II

This stage is characterized by more obvious cognitive dysfunction. The person will become less fluent. Often he will begin to misunderstand conversation. The ability to fully understand the punch line of a joke may be lost. As the disease evolves, information in newspaper and magazine articles is at first misinterpreted, and, finally, not understood. Television shows become progressively incomprehensible. This results in a slow withdrawal from communication activities such as television, radio, periodicals, and newspapers.

In this stage, difficulties with checkbooks and financial management become obvious. There is a more subtle loss in the ability to plan ahead. The individual also becomes more self-centered and insensitive to the needs and feelings of others. He or she may function quite well in many other ways, but the degree of supervision over his or her activities must be intensified. All of the symptoms of Stage I worsen and new symptoms appear:

Agnosia—the inability to recognize objects that should be familiar either by visual, auditory, or touch-related (tactile) stimulation. In visual agnosia a person may not recognize the difference between a face and a hat. He or she may not recognize food. Although there is nothing wrong with his or her vision, he or she is unable to intellectually recognize the significance of the object, its purpose, and its intent.

Apraxia—the inability to perform an act even though the motor ability to perform that act is left intact. Even though there is no paralysis or motor dysfunction that prevents him or her from doing so, the demented person may be unable to perform a simple task like folding a piece of paper. It is as though the command for action cannot be transferred from the brain to the hands for action.

Alexia—difficulty with reading and, finally, loss of the ability to read.

Agraphia—difficulty and, ultimately, the loss of the ability to write.

Aphasia—difficulty in the ability to speak and understand language, both written and spoken.

In Stage II, the demented person may become restless at night. He or she may fixate on an idea or response and it may dominate conversation. He or she may get lost intermittently, experiencing difficulty in finding the bathroom when visiting a friend or family member's home. As the disease progresses, he or she may not be able to locate the bathroom in his or her own home. His or her gait appears stiff and slow. Spontaneous movements about his or her face, such as smiling and laughing, decrease considerably. In the final days of Stage II, he or she may have to be reminded to perform the activities of daily living that we all do without reminder—brushing teeth, bathing, and dressing.

STAGES III AND IV

As Stage III begins, the dementia victim's disability is obvious. Orientation to time and place is clearly defective. The patient may be unable to identify familiar faces and persons, even family members. He or she becomes so unsure, particularly in social settings, that complete withdrawal is the general rule. Memory is very poor, but memory of the distant past is not necessarily affected and may, in fact, remain with great clarity until death. He or she may exhibit bizarre behavior, such as urinating in the corner of a room or wearing clothes inappropriately. He or she may wear underwear for days at a time without changing.

As multiple examples of bizarre behavior evidence themselves, the terminal stage begins. It is at this time that the disease has its fullest expression. Some professionals refer to this as Stage IV, while others view it as an extension of the third stage.

The dementia victim becomes apathetic and withdrawn. He or she may sleep the majority of the daytime hours or may have his or her sleep rhythm significantly disrupted, so that he or she is up all night and sleeps only portions of the day. Night wandering becomes much more common. At this point he or she may fail to recognize his or her closest friend or family member and may have a significant amount of anxiety when placed in the presence of this "stranger."

In Stage IV, persons with dementia become unable to care for themselves. Speech and motor abilities are progressively lost. Speech deteriorates to a nonfluent state with single-word answers. Vocabulary is limited to as few as six words and, ultimately, verbal communication ceases.

Anxiety and frightened behavior appear for no apparent reason. Occasionally, combativeness may occur due to the high level of anxiety. The ability to smile is gone forever. As the demented person nears death, he or she becomes bedridden and totally dependent on others for care. Most frequently, death by pneumonia, urinary tract infection, or choking on food or vomit follows as a complication of being bedridden. In many cases, the person lapses into a coma from which he or she never awakens.

Frequently, when demented persons are moved to nursing homes or other institutions, their confusion dramatically worsens for a time, due to the change in location from familiar to unfamiliar surroundings. This confusion is often misunderstood by the caregiver and blamed on medications. Infection and pain are common internal stimuli that result in a temporary worsening of the demented patient's condition. When the infection is eliminated, the demented person may return to his or her "normal" condition.

Dementia may appear for the first time in an apparently mentally well individual while he or she is in the hospital for treatment of an unrelated condition. Your loved one may go to the hospital for a hernia operation and do well the first night. But on the second or third night in the hospital, he or she may become progressively more confused. This can be the first clue that a loved one is having difficulty with his or her brain and may be developing a dementing illness.

When Dementia is Diagnosed

- Try not to make changes in the home once the diagnosis of dementia has been established. This includes arrangements of furniture and other articles, painting, etc.
- Demented patients should not be moved from relative to relative for respite care, as this will tend to strongly disorient him or her.
- At night, when visual cues decrease, disorientation, anxiety, and sometimes combativeness increase. Leave a light on in the bedroom and in the bathroom. This night light assists with orientation if the person awakens. Be sure that familiar items are around the person in bed. Lighting should be bright enough so that it does not cast unfamiliar shadows.
- Be particularly cautious of new medications. They frequently make behavior worse. The worst offenders are those that are used for high blood pressure, sleep, sedation, and anxiety.
- Early in the disease, keep the patient as active as possible. Take him or her on short trips to familiar places and encourage familiar activities. Select a familiar hobby and encourage the care recipient to expand on that hobby. If he or she does not have a hobby, a small garden or greenhouse with simple plants may be the answer.
- In order to avoid sleep problems, use the bedroom only for sleeping. Discourage daytime naps and the consumption of caffeine. Adhere to a strict schedule, arising each morning at the same time, preferably early, with no allowance for "sleeping in" or napping, in order to maintain the regimen and rigidity of the sleep schedule.

Taking Care of the Caregiver

Caregiving can be dangerous to your health if not entered into with adequate preparation and knowledge. The process of providing intensive care can affect the health status of the very one who needs to remain healthy.

Dementia is a family illness. The patient requires constant care and attention. Normal childhood development, including the evolution of progressive independence, is reversed. The demented person instead regresses to total dependence. To meet this challenge and to provide appropriate, loving care, caregivers must be familiar with their own needs, convictions, inner thoughts, and abilities to recognize the unfamiliar emotional responses that will arise during caregiving.

The caregiver travels a tumultuous emotional journey. Identification and management of its signposts and detours are essential to the well-being of the caregiver. Denial, initially encompassing fear and sadness, anger, depression, guilt, and resentment, must be recognized and overcome. The ability to identify and deal with those emotions determines the success that the caregiver, friends, and family members will have in avoiding illness themselves.

Recent studies of caregivers and their health complaints show that during the first 16 to 18 months of caregiving the caregiver is enthusiastic, dedicated, and energetic and has few or no physical complaints. As the caregiver attempts to meet the care recipient's increasing physical and emotional demands in months 16 through 24, the caregiver him- or herself begins to have complaints of chronic pain, poor sleep maintenance, and a variety of other symptoms.

In the second and third years of caregiving, these symptoms intensify and expand, and the number of physician office visits on the part of the caregiver increases. Complaints on the part of the caregiver may include insomnia, headache, fatigue, high blood pressure, back pain, depression, unexplained weight loss, and accentuation of any preexisting cardiac, gastrointestinal, and neurological symptoms. After three years, caregivers generally suffer a significant decline in health and may seek psychiatric or psychological care on a regular basis.

The first step in meeting the caregiving challenge lies in realizing that the caregiver cannot be effective unless he or she loves and respects him- or herself. Confidence in dealing with others demands a certain inner self-respect. It encompasses a willingness to share that self-love with another without being afraid of losing control or being hurt. It involves a certain primacy of self-care, self-help, and self-interest.

The caregiver has to recognize that there is an uncertain brevity in all our lives that requires and demands caring for oneself first. Time for solitude away from the ill person and time for self-pleasure, including entertainment, friends, hobbies, and exercise, must be guarded if he or she is to remain an effective caregiver. All-encompassing dedication to the ill person is destructive in the long-term, both to the care recipient and to the caregiver.

Bad news is never welcome. We never want to hear that someone we know is gravely ill, dying, or dead. Our front-line emotional self-defense is the initial refusal to accept that news. A corollary is the constant hope that recovery will occur at some time in the future. Denial is our temporary method of coping. It protects us from the shock of bad news and gives us time to deal on an emotional level with unwanted news.

Denial that persists can be disastrous for the person doing the denying, as well as for the person who is the object of the denial. Ignoring a loved one's memory loss or disorientation may result in injury. It prevents the meeting of real needs. Examples of denial include:

"There is nothing wrong with you (the care recipient) and everything would be better if you would just go out, be sociable, and make friends."

"Since Dad died, you just sit around and talk to me. You're just trying to get me to pay more attention to you."

Later, after the onset of dementia is obvious, denial may take the form of a continual search for new treatments, research specialists geographically removed from home, experimental unproven drugs from outside the country, or miracle-cure health foods. This hopefulness often results in a devastating expenditure of financial resources and physical and emotional energies. Worse, it denies the real needs of the demented person: caring, structuring, nurturing, and loving.

It is essential that caregivers confront and acknowledge the disease, accept the diagnosis, and deal with the fact that nothing can be done to reverse the onset of dementia. Be cognizant of your own feelings; those feelings will influence your relationships with others, including the care recipient, your immediate family, and friends. You must attempt to understand others' feelings as well your own.

Try to understand why you are feeling a certain way. Explore the reasons for negative feelings so that the same emotions will not reappear later when a similar situation arises, blocking a more positive approach.

If necessary, seek out support group help or psychological counseling to help sort out negative feelings.

Demented persons evoke a variety of emotions in those around them, particularly the caregiver. There may be continual frustration because of memory lapses or public embarrassment because of antisocial or inappropriate behavior and the inability of a demented patient to care for his or her own personal hygiene and needs. This anger may be expressed in a variety of ways. A caregiver may ignore the demented person's needs by allowing him or her to remain soiled with feces because "it serves him right." He or she may chastise the care recipient with the threat of "no visitors" or "no food" because of the inability to remember simple chores that should have been performed but were not.

Frequently, anger is directed at physicians and other health professionals because they "do not care," do not spend sufficient time with the patient, or do not return calls as quickly as the caregiver might expect. Nursing home placement frequently triggers the release of pent-up anger as the caregiver attempts to deal with his or her feelings of guilt.

When anger is not expressed, it is internalized and may appear later in self-destructive behaviors, such as drinking, substance abuse, and overeating. Somatic complaints, such as ulcers, headaches and backaches, and colitis, and psychosomatic illnesses and neuroses, including anxiety and depression, may result.

Perhaps more than any other disease, dementia intimately and perilously involves the caregiver and the care recipient. Persons with dementia have no insight into their illnesses, and as they lose cognitive function they also lose the ability to understand the emotions of those around them. Relatives who see the care recipient infrequently may not understand the stress that the caregiver bears. The fact is that family members who are not actively involved in a loved one's care have little insight into the problems that occur day in and day out, 24 hours a day. They will not understand the emotional range exhibited by the caregiver.

The caregiver will have feelings of isolation and abandonment, particularly if siblings or children avoid assuming responsibility for the demented person. To avoid misunderstandings, the caregiver must, at the very beginning of the illness, communicate with other family members the degree of the illness and its prognosis, as well as its symptoms. Family members who provide respite for full-time caregivers may experience a revelation in dealing with their loved ones.

At some point, all caregivers need someone to talk to. Do not hesitate to seek out a friend, minister, counselor, or health professional. Loneliness, despair, a sense of betrayal, and fear need to be expressed and discussed. Generally they are at the root of anger.

Dementia takes its toll on caregivers, friends, and family members. It causes illness in caregivers, disrupts families, and produces a spectrum of emotions that is rarely seen in other illnesses. Anticipation of those feelings and learning responses that assist in their management is the basis for avoiding illness and distress in the caregiver.

Live for yourself, and live one day at a time.

The Caregivers' Bible

- Maintain social contacts and as many social activities as possible.
- Formally, and in writing, schedule respite time for yourself on a daily or weekly basis. Even a few minutes a day can make a difference in your outlook. Stick to that schedule.
- Involve other relatives in the care of the care recipient early on, including multiple-day care over weekends or holidays.
- Do not martyr yourself. No one should expect to provide all care every day without help. If possible, get a job or activity away from home for periods of time.
- Make sure that children and siblings understand the disease. Let them assume caregiving duties for short periods so that they can experience first hand the stress you experience as caregiver. They, too, will suffer doubt, denial, guilt, and anger, and the fury may be directed at you.
- Guilt and anger are normal emotions. Recognize them for what they are and avoid acting on them. Anger usually accompanies a sense of guilt.
- The incidence of headache, insomnia, backache, or other physical complaints during caregiving can be stress-related, stemming from unresolved anger, guilt, and/or depression. Nearly all caregivers are physically affected by the care recipient's illness. Face that fact and accept it. To remain an effective caregiver, you must take time out for yourself.

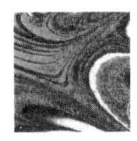

Profile

"Daisy" grew up in a family of eight siblings in a rural community in the South. After finishing her schooling she moved to Philadelphia, was successful in the job market, married, and had two sons, now 31 and 14, and a daughter, now 25.

For 19 years, Daisy has been responsible for the care of one or both of her parents. There have been many problems as a result of chronic health conditions, as well as conflict among Daisy's siblings over financial and property matters.

Daisy's mother was mentally ill and was hospitalized at Florida State Hospital while Daisy was a young girl. While her mother had a rough life there, Daisy says, she was helped and "did beautifully." However, her mother never overcame her obsession with the belief that she had a baby that needed—but was being deprived of—her care and attention. This idea remained with her mother for the rest of her life. She was also a diabetic.

In 1971, Daisy moved her mother to Philadelphia to live with her in her home. Daisy was 32; her mother was 60. This arrangement worked well. Then in 1988, Daisy was forced to move back to her childhood home with her younger son and her mother, to live with her father and provide care for him. Her sister had attempted to care for her father, but ran into so many difficulties with other relatives that she left. Daisy should have been forewarned.

The move was very hard on Daisy's mother. It meant "going back" to a life she had left 30 years before.

In 1988, Daisy started building a home on the family property. When it was completed, she moved her parents and her younger son into the new house. Soon after moving into her new home, Daisy's mother's condition worsened. She became bedridden and, six months later, died. Daisy's father had suffered several strokes and was hardly aware of the move. He has since had to have both legs amputated.

Daisy's older son moved down from Philadelphia to help Daisy with his grandfather's care. He gave up his own interests and his life to come and take on this responsibility. Daisy says, "He has done a tremendous job."

Daisy resents the fact that her three brothers living in the community don't find the time to visit or help. In fact, the family has been in and out of court with disputes over the property and her right to build there. Her brothers contend that when Daisy and her sisters moved away, they gave up their rights to the family home.

The brothers have initiated abuse investigations with the Department of Health and Rehabilitative Services accused Daisy of not allowing them to visit. Daisy has never gone to court with her complaints, but a judge finally required that the brother who has guardianship rights contribute from their father's Social Security check toward the cost of his care.

Daisy said the fighting has been difficult for her, physically and emotionally. One doctor recommended nursing home care for her father. "I told the doctor that my whole idea was to come here and care for him. He had asked us never to put him in a nursing home," Daisy says. "He sacrificed a lot for us, and I believe I owe it to him."

Daisy sees the caregiving experience as having changed her life in every way. "There is only one way to care for your parents: to believe in God and take your burden to Him. He has made me strong."

Her four sisters call and encourage Daisy. "They're beautiful," she says. "If someone is willing to care for two parents, all the other family members should be in their corner."

Caring and Grieving

Karen Ring, M.S.W., L.C.S.W.

I was 7 years old when I had my first experience with death and grief. I was at the funeral of my great-grandmother, Bubba Chelpanoff. She lay in a casket in her living room, the casket now replacing the bed she had died in a few days earlier. Everyone loved Bubba Chelpanoff and her daughters had taken care of her throughout her illness. I overheard my mother saying that Bubba had struggled during her last few weeks. She slept sitting up with her eyes open, fearful that if she closed them she would never wake up again.

Her house was filled with Russian Orthodox prayers, the smell of burning incense and candles, huge arrangements of flowers, and crying friends and family members dressed in black. As the casket was to be closed and Bubba taken to the cemetery for burial, my mother fainted, overwhelmed with the grief of losing her grandmother. Smelling salts revived her.

Weeks later, lying in bed on a stormy Saturday morning, I played funeral. With my sheets and blanket, I created the cemetery where Bubba Chelpanoff was buried. My fingers climbed the hill, becoming the men, women, and children who loved her. They cried and chanted an old Orthodox hymn.

We all share in the universal experience of grief. There are common themes and understandings that require no explanation. We are a community of grievers. There are also differences in our grief that another could never imagine or know. Our grief is uniquely our own by virtue of living our own personal life. We stand isolated and alone. Death and grief may seem like the final reward for the many long hours of giving, caring, and loving one another. Whether we give out of love or obligation or both, caregiving simultaneously holds losses and gains.

The reality is that death and loss are a part of the fabric of existence, no matter how much we ignore, avoid, or try to tear out this basic part of our lives. What is important is how we respond to loss. And this is what grief is: our response to loss, to change, to transition, to death, to confusion, to being overtaken by the shifting of the reality of our lives.

Caregivers have the potential for being grief filled. Grief does not begin when the care recipient dies. Grief begins with the caregiver's own loss of time, freedom, and privacy. It begins when you see your mother aging and you can not seem to tolerate her forgetfulness. It begins when you can not be your "daddy's little girl" anymore because you are taking care of him more than he is taking care of you. Grief begins when you miss the quiet talks and walks with your husband because he has suffered a stroke, or when you realize that your sister is not just sick, but dying. Grief begins when you realize that neither you nor your life will ever be the same again. And grief begins when you are a child and lose someone you love for the first time.

At no time in our life is grief felt so overwhelmingly as when we take on the responsibility of caring for another person because of their diminishing life or ability to care for themselves due to aging, disability, or illness. Not only do we have to deal with our own grief, but most likely the person we are caring for is also experiencing a loss. Grief immediately and unmercifully makes us face the inevitable outcome for ourselves and others: death.

It is a very different experience to live with grief and loss as opposed to studying, analyzing, or writing about it. As you read this chapter on grieving, remember that there are no experts on your grief. There are no rules that you have to follow to be "okay." Use this information as a structure to hang onto during those tumultuous times when you seem lost. Allow grief to be its own experience, your own teacher about life and death. This chapter is a sharing of ideas and the knowledge of many people who are interested in grief and who have reported their findings; it is not meant to negate your own knowledge. It will be important as you read to know your own feelings and experience, and to voice the unsaid truth of your grief. Take along your courage as you care for yourself and others who are grieving.

Grief Is...

grief/'gref/ n [MEgref,fr.OF, heavy, grave] 1: emotional suffering caused by or as if by bereavement

bereave/bi-'rev/[ME bereaven, fr. be-+reafian to rob] 1: to deprive esp. by death: strip, dispossess 2: to take away- be reave ment

Grief is our reaction to loss, the loss of someone or something to which we are emotionally attached. It is the feeling of being robbed of life and our relationship to that life. It is the feeling of losing a part of ourselves. In reality, grief is not just one reaction. It is a continuous process of a multitude of expectable and unexpected reactions to an external event that seems to tear apart our internal being.

Our grief is a universal, natural, adaptive process necessary to let go of what was, and to be ready for what is to come. Everybody grieves, not just about death, but about all kinds of losses. Most of us carry around within us unexpressed grief accumulated from years of minor and major losses. This unexplored, unfinished grief can come to the surface to join forces with our current loss, making the already devastating experience overwhelming.

There are various theories or ways of looking at grief. It can be seen as a crisis, an illness, a stage of development, or a transition. It may be all of these, because grief is complex, affecting us and others in many areas at the same time.

The four major areas where our grief is played out are the physical, psychological, social, and spiritual.

Physically, grief can stress our bodies and lower our immune system. It can manifest itself as crying, tearfulness, shortness of breath, chest tightness, heart palpitations, anxiety, exhaustion and fatigue, sleep disturbances, weight loss or gain, anorexia, gastrointestinal disorders, nervousness, restlessness, sighing, agitation, changes in sexual behavior and interest, decreased energy and motivation, loss of pleasure, or almost any physical symptom. These symptoms are not unusual, and most people experience some of them.

Psychologically, grief affects our feelings, thoughts, and attitudes. Most people suffer from shock, denial, self-pity, yearning, anger, relief, guilt, anxiety, panic, mental confusion, depression, sadness, acceptance, and hope, at varying times. Socially, our behavior with our partners, family, children, church, or community is just as deeply affected. Our social interaction can run the gamut from offering us support and stability during a difficult time to being a source of pain and dysfunction. The ability to start and continue relationships is diminished. Social withdrawal may occur and people may treat us differently. All of this is expected.

Finally, grief can reaffirm or destroy the very foundation of our spiritual beliefs about what life is and what it means to us. Finding meaning in the experience of loss is a key in the grieving process.

How you express your grief is based on your own individual and unique perception of your world and your loss. Grief is necessary to help you adapt and move on to your new life, and it can be awful. Our life will never be the same as it was before our loss. The old life has passed away. It may be better or worse, but it will be different. Without death and loss there can be no new life.

The cultural context of our grief is important as we look at both our own expectations of how we grieve and what society expects of us. In most cultures, people grieve a person's death and also believe that the person who dies continues to exist in some way beyond death. Cultures usually differ widely in how loss is defined and in the appropriateness of its expression. In the United States, despite its wide range of ethnic diversity, the white, male, Anglo-Saxon, Protestant mentality prevails. The expectation is one of self-control and of suffering in silence. This may be a particularly difficult expectation for people of other cultures who want to assimilate into the American culture. The extreme reactions to grief can become muted and abnormal.

In our culture, we have a fear of anger and hostility. Many feel guilty for even having these feelings, while in other cultures anger and aggression are expected and expressed through ritual. So we tend to minimize and deny our grief reactions. In some cases, people's losses are not even acknowledged or, if they are, there is an expectation of a compressed and unrealistic recovery time.

Because many people are uncomfortable with grief and seem lost when it comes to helping or supporting one another, the community may isolate the grieving family during times of loss. Death, illness, and aging have become more remote as we have segregated the ill and elderly. In the past, symbolic activities and rituals have supported and directed the bereaved. Now, however, their use has diminished and isolation has increased.

The American family has also gone through changes over the last few decades that affect its ability to handle grief. Families have become less extended and more nuclear, putting the burden of caregiving and dealing with loss on fewer members. Many families find that they are not able to meet all of their own needs, especially with the increased emotional involvement of fewer members. In other cultures with larger, extended families, the emotional intensity of relationships is usually less, and more widely dispersed. In cases of larger families, in the United States they are usually geographically unavailable to provide physical assistance due to increased mobility and family separation. Even in the best of times, some families are dysfunctional and there may be ambivalence and higher levels of unresolved grief, making it necessary for some members to express their grief through withdrawal from the situation.

Perhaps one of the most difficult cultural aspects to overcome—and one that has also been integrated into our own personal self-image—is the American belief of personal mastery and control over life. As a nation we see ourselves as strong, capable, and able to handle anything. When we are in grief, the reality may be that we feel weak, lost, and victimized. The horrible truth may be that we cannot do this alone and that we need help from others. Americans are known internationally for their sometimes over-exuberant positiveness about life, their continual search for youth, and optimistic attitudes and behavior. This is not so much a criticism as an observation that there is another side of life that must be dealt with. Grief throws us into it head on, whether we acknowledge it or not.

Personality characteristics and coping styles also factor heavily into what grief is for us individually. Our own level of awareness about loss and death, as well as our own past experiences, will help us define how we handle our own losses and the losses of others. Awareness and expression of our feelings and needs during times of distress will influence our grief. In general, our attitude about living will have an effect on our attitude about dying and loss. Practical implications such as our health, education, age, gender, and financial situation are also important.

In our culture, men are not expected to express grief through tears. Sometimes we can be more fearful of our financial resources running out before death occurs than of the actual death itself. A myriad of personal and collective influences make grief uniquely our own.

Normal Grief Reactions

In your role as caregiver, knowledge and understanding of the emotional reactions and processes of grief in the aging, ill, or dying care recipient will be necessary in order for you to provide adequate emotional care, support, and comfort to that person. Awareness of grief will also be helpful in your role as caregiver because you, too, will experience grief. Grief reactions are an up-and-down phenomenon and rarely run a straight course. Grief "attacks"—waves of grief that come over a person, sometimes for no explainable reason—are frequent. It will be helpful to look at the following reactions as simplified, but, in reality, they combine and intersect with one another at various times to become unique to each person and very complex.

Usually the first experience of loss is shock. Like our bodies, our minds protect us from overwhelming pain, and we are numb. Confidence is shaken. Denial is another first line of defense and the bereaved is filled with disbelief that the loss has happened. Shock and denial may come and go, but until the shaken internal and external worlds have been given some order, the events precipitating the loss will be reviewed over and over again. Life seems to be lived in slow motion. Adjustment to this new reality may take some time, especially if an illness or disease is diagnosed. Denial for some may last through the death experience.

After some of the shock has worn off, yearning for the lost person or life becomes paramount in the mind of the griever. The bereaved thinks about the lost loved one or life obsessively and may go searching in his or her own way. An aching woundedness and emptiness accompany the deep feelings and sense of loss. The yearning is not only psychological but physical, since the touch and presence of who or what has been lost is missed.

Sometimes the grieving person will hear, see, smell, or feel the presence of a person who has died. Auditory and visual hallucinations are not uncommon, and dreams may contain interactions with the deceased. There may be a yearning for an earlier time or a special place. Yearning and searching are ways of trying to make sense out of the loss and eventually will end, because of the fruitlessness of the search and the resulting pain.

Self-pity may be one of first feelings that returns after the numbness wears off. There is a sense of isolation and a belief that this tragedy has happened only to you. The grieving person finds it difficult to recognize anything but his or her own pain. In times of grief and loss in a family, this particular reaction can bring added loss when the expectation is that others will be there to provide comfort. Instead, others, too, seem caught up in their own loss. Self-pity is natural and closely connected to the anger one feels at loss. The caregiver needs to allow the grieving person to have self-pity and then slowly encourage him or her to look or reach outside of him- or herself and reassess some of the good aspects of life.

Anger is a natural consequence of being deprived of something or someone valued. Anger can be manifested as irritability, frustration, intolerance, annoyance, bitterness, and sarcasm. Some people provoke arguments and may even lash out physically. The angry, bereaved person can be angry at doctors, relatives, friends, the person who died, a disease, caregivers, God, and him- or herself. In our culture, anger is the most acceptable way for men to express grief, while women usually express grief through tears.

In both cases, it might be beneficial to identify what the person is really feeling. Anger needs to be encouraged as long as no one is being emotionally or physically abused. There can be a fine line, but as caregiver it will be important for you to determine what that line is.

Relief is the feeling one has when a great ordeal has been ended. For the aging, ill, or dying person, this may occur when some struggle with pain or disease has been overcome. For the caregiver, relief may be felt when the elderly person dies, especially after years of caregiving. There is a gladness that life can get back to normal and that there will be some rest and freedom. Exhaustion and fatigue may set in. To have relief does not diminish the care one had for the person but it can be guilt producing for the survivors.

Guilt is the cognitive and emotional response to believing that there was something you could have done or not done to have staved off the loss. There may be appropriate guilt, because we are not perfect and there are probably things we could have done or said that might have helped. Maybe not. If guilt is appropriate, then we need to forgive ourselves, knowing that we fall short of our expectations and standards.

When we are in grief, we tend to look at the negative and exaggerate it. A dying person may blame him- or herself for causing an illness when in reality there is nothing that he or she could have done. Taking the guilt or blame is another way of somehow gaining control over an uncontrollable event, loss, or death. Many people blame themselves as a means of bringing order to this chaos.

Anxiety, panic, and fear are related reactions to loss. Anxiety has to do more with an unknown, undefinable fear and sense of insecurity about what life will be like with this debilitating illness or unavoidable change. The inability to control seemingly out-of-control events in life can lead to panic. These reactions may exhibit themselves in sleeplessness and nightmares, compulsive or impulsive behaviors, and frequent illness. If there has been a major loss then there is fear that another tragedy may occur, because the world can no longer be trusted. A sense of powerlessness, helplessness, and worry prevail and the need to control may increase.

Confusion exists because the order and sense of self have been altered. An aging parent may be confused due to the new living arrangements of moving in with his or her adult child. Because of a shift in identity, emotions change daily and there is an inability to make decisions because thinking has been affected. Assertion may come out of fear. Confusion may be mistaken for ambivalence since, in grief, people will have conflicting feelings. This, too, is normal.

Regression is common not only in the aging and sick but also in anyone who is experiencing deep feelings of loss. Stripped of our appropriate masks, manners, and societal expectations, grief can take us back to that lost and frightened inner child who still lives inside of us and is at the core of our personality. Grief can make us feel like a helpless, needy child, unable to identify or articulate the extent of the injury. Childish behavior in a grieving person needs to be met with compassion and encouragement rather than admonishment or disgust.

Depression can be a constructive aspect of the grief process. It cushions us from too much emotional shock and minimizes incoming stress. Since our energy level is low, it allows for rest and healing to occur. It also may protect us from making decisions. Feelings of sadness, abandonment, and despair heighten. Physical symptoms may occur, such as insomnia or increased sleeping, poor appetite or overeating, and increased or frequent illness. The person who is depressed may neglect his or her appearance and withdraw from friends, activities, and hobbies.

Depression can turn destructive if the person begins using alcohol or other drugs to self-medicate the emotional pain of grief. He or she may even consider suicide. If suicide is suspected, ask the bereaved if he or she has been frequently thinking of killing him- or herself and ask if there is a plan to do so. The idea of suicide needs to be openly addressed, since more and more people in our country are viewing it as an alternative. Suicide can be an avoidance of pain, an attempt to gain control and speed up the process of dying, or, in the case of survivors, an attempt to be reunited with lost loved ones. If there are any doubts about how to handle this possibility it may be necessary to call in a mental health professional.

It is very difficult to determine when the care recipient is suffering from clinical or chronic depression versus acute depression due to a normal grief reaction. Grief and depression are similar in feelings, moods, and behavior, but the main difference is that the depressed person's thinking or understanding is distorted. Negative perceptions are persistent, intense, of long duration, and are usually self-condemning.

The grieving individual feels sad and can change to more normal moods on a daily basis. A depressed person feels sadness and anger that is directed toward him- or herself.

A grieving person will express anger appropriate to the situation, whereas a depressed person may express anger through rage or deny being angry at all, even though it seems that to get angry would be the normal thing to do.

A grieving person will be able to enjoy pleasure and respond to warmth and reassurance, while the depressed person rarely enjoys anything pleasurable and is unresponsive to others and their assistance. The depressed person feels a decrease in self-esteem, seeing him- or herself as worthless at times, and may harbor feelings of irrational guilt. It becomes increasingly difficult to empathize with the depressed person because nothing that is done or said makes a difference in his or her negative view of the future, which contains no hope or acceptance of fate.

True sadness is a sincere missing of what one is losing or has lost. Without feeling worthless or incapable, there is an emptiness that is acknowledged and felt. Sadness is intermingled with the other reactions and can be felt through the body in sighing and fatigue. There is a realization that some things in life just are not as important anymore. In the sadness there is a hope for survival.

In grief there is a time when acceptance emerges and, more and more, the reality of the loss is faced. Some of the other reactions begin to leave, and what remains is just hurt and missing the loved one or object of loss. If the grieving person is in the dying process, acceptance may mark the beginning of peace and a readiness for the unknown mystery of what awaits beyond death to unfold. For the survivor, joys are once again experienced, as well as a renewed trust in oneself.

Hope in oneself and life will begin when the survivor is able to enjoy something again without the painful thought of the loved one. There is a sense of healing and accomplishment at having survived the loss.

Feelings of confidence, independence, and peace help create a new life and an encouragement to go on with it.

At resolution, the bereaved is able to say goodbye to the loved one and live on with the loss. It is acknowledged that the person who was lost continues on as a part of the inner self through memories. The grieving person begins to reinvest in new relationships and activities, deciding to develop a new trust in the world.

Anticipatory Grief

Anticipatory grief is the normal grief people begin to feel with the possibility of the impending death of a loved one or when they first realize that their own illness will be terminal. Anticipatory grief includes many of the symptoms one experiences following a loss. The dying care recipient experiences anticipatory grief, too, along with the family and caregiver. Not only do the grievers grieve for the loss of their future life, but also for their past and current losses. Especially in debilitating diseases such as dementia and Alzheimer's disease, the family and caregiver mourn the loss of the person they used to know, as well as the person who will be unable to participate in future plans and dreams. The current losses, perhaps the loss of logical thinking or control over one's own life, are also grieved.

This process of grieving prior to the death of an individual allows for the gradual adapting to the reality of the loss and the changing assumptions about it. Anticipatory grief allows for the unfinished business of saying and doing things while there is still time left.

There are difficulties inherent in this type of grief, notwithstanding the advantages anticipatory grief has over a sudden unforeseen death. Conflicts arise, such as becoming closer to the dying person through heightened concern and care, while needing to separate from him or her in an attempt to adjust to the consequences of death. The caregiver may imagine what life will be like without the care recipient and then feel that they have betrayed the person.

Trying to take care of the dying person's needs and care versus trying to take care of oneself may be a constant source of conflict. Theses are just a few of the complications that anticipatory grief produces as the inevitability of loss and death emerge. For the dying person, the family, and the caregiver, the balance is to see anticipatory grief as necessary while enjoying the remaining time of living as fully as possible.

Complicated, Abnormal, and Unresolved Grief

The natural process of grieving can be absent, prolonged, or distorted in many ways. Individuals and families prone to complicated grief can be identified through some common characteristics.
Some of the factors to take into consideration are:

- a history of substance abuse (alcohol, drugs, cigarettes, food)
- social isolation and no support system
- recent multiple losses of any kind
- unresolved grief from previous losses
- lack of time for grief expression
- overly dependent or ambivalent relationships with dying or deceased persons
- persistent denial of the dying process
- long-term caregiving
- a history of suicides
- rigid religiosity (the belief that all life-threatening illnesses need to be healed)
- a history of depression or mental illness.

Grief can become complicated due to the nature of the illness or death, the caregiver's or survivor's psychological traits and relationship with the care recipient, and the inability to express feelings related to the loss.

Absent grief occurs when the bereaved person experiences no emotion or reaction to the loss. Shock and denial are strong and continuous. Absent grief should not be confused with grief that a person feels but is unable to verbally express.

Distorted grief is manifested when the grieving person minimizes the emotional reactions as unimportant or unnecessary. Displaced grief is another distorted or conflicted reaction. It is usually expressed as exaggerated anger and guilt, focused toward self and others. In these types of reactions only parts of the various emotions are allowed to surface and be expressed.

An example of converted grief is when emotions are expressed through the body, or somaticized. Headaches, backaches, stomach problems, muscular tension, and numerous other maladies may surface. Health problems, which are more frequent in the bereaved, may be the single most apparent indicator of unresolved grief. Older people, in particular, tend to manifest their grief through illness.

Replaced grief may be another way of diminishing the feeling of loss. The person may take on more activities to stay busy or quickly get involved in another relationship as a means of avoiding the pain that working through grief requires.

Chronic grief is the continuous, intense grief that was felt appropriately at the initial time of loss but is still being exhibited after the passage of time. The bereaved person seems stuck in the early phases of the grief reactions as if the loss had just happened. Yearning for the lost person or aspect of life still continues and the person cannot or is unwilling to let go. Sometimes the grief will not be properly dealt with by the bereaved until months or years have passed.

Chronic grief is characteristic of people who made an overly large investment in the lost object of their affection and love. The holding on may also be due to past unresolved conflicts or a dysfunctional relationship that has not yet been addressed. Many people are unable to develop close or lasting relationships because of this lack of resolution.

Complicated grief is usually a result of avoidance or denial of the feelings surrounding loss, either self-imposed or imposed by others. Grief is something that is not "gotten over" but, rather, something that is lived through. Resolution of that grief may take years. It is a variable process with no specific time frame. As long as the bereaved person is able to function socially or exhibits no harmful or pathological behavior, then grief is not abnormal. The same holds true for the elderly dying person, although some circumstances will call for more sensitivity to the person's overall dying process. However, when a person experiences complicated grief, it may be necessary to seek professional help.

Aging as Loss

Aunt Miriam called last week from Pittsburgh to report that Uncle Jimmy had died. She also told me about Uncle Joe's deteriorating knees and his fluctuations between depression and overdoing it. His disability and early retirement from being an active milkman is driving her crazy. Aunt Miriam and Uncle Joe raised four kids together, and his 14-hour milk delivery day gave them little shared time. Now that he is home all the time, adapting to the change and being with a very unhappy person is sometimes more than Aunt Miriam can bear. She continues to wait on his every need as she has done for the last 38 years. To make matters worse, many of his friends are now being given some dark diagnoses *t*hemselves. Aunt Miriam ended her telephone call to me with this prophetic warning: "Don't believe what anyone tells you about how great getting old is. All our friends are getting sick and dying. We ache and are worried how we'll manage the money. Getting old is sad... it's terrible." Later, after hanging up the phone, I wondered if my life will come to this, too.

Aging, among other things, can mean experiencing grief due to both physical loss and symbolic loss. In physical loss, we may lose the use of a leg or part of our body, but we also lose symbolically. There may be losses of independence, control, and security, which will disrupt a person's self-image. Some believe that aging begins at middle age with an inevitable, gradual diminishment of vitality. To stave off the outer evidence of aging we may cover it up with hair color, wigs, dental work, or facelifts-all in an attempt to slow down our movement toward old age.

In our country, aging is seen as a loss of youth, something to be avoided at all costs. Perhaps the demise of old wise men and crones began as more people began to search for wisdom at the Fountain of Youth. Whatever the cultural implications of this shift may be, the fact remains that grieving for these partial losses of aging is considered shameful and avoided by some older persons.

People are usually aware of the slow changes happening as they age. As we age, losses manifest themselves, physically and through the senses. There is a loss of hair and teeth, skin changes, and we experience slower healing. Sight and hearing diminish and we feel tired and cold more often. The possibility of a fall or stroke can cause fear of dependence or of being a burden on the family.

Physical changes give way to social changes and losses. With decreased mobility, there is less possibility of visiting old friends and more possibility of losing peers to distance or death. This can exacerbate the psychological losses that are also felt during aging. A person's sense of autonomy and independence as a capable human being diminishes, and the way a family and community treat the elderly may reinforce personal losses through loneliness and isolation. More and more energy is used to adapt to the deterioration of the body, and a minimum daily routine is the highest goal for the day's events. Fear of illnesses, diseases, and future losses can also come into consciousness for the elderly person.

In trying to prolong youth and good health, more people are living longer than ever before, but they are living with an array of chronic, debilitative, degenerative diseases that have made aging itself into a kind of dying. With the onset of illness, the aging person begins to take on the role of the sick person. Health is now being lost. Other losses such as predictability and consistency may ensue. If still working at a career or meaningful activity, inability to continue may also affect self-worth.

Loss of dreams and hopes for the future may become more evident as efforts to deal with poor health become a priority. As health declines, outside or family assistance may bring a loss of privacy. Moving in order to receive caregiving and the subsequent loss of familiar housing and possessions can be a traumatic, remarkable event in an aging person's life. If the aging person was a caregiver, the shift to the role of care recipient will be another adjustment and loss to contend with, perhaps throughout the now-shifted caregiving relationship. Roles, tasks, and identity are eroding. Finally, the money spent on caring for the aging person, along with rising health care costs, can be anxiety producing for the care recipient and family members.

If we look at the aging person's dilemma, we can easily see life as a fruitless ending, a despairing outcome to a long held- onto life. According to Erik Erikson's psychological theory, a person moves into the final stage of life by reassessing, accepting and integrating who he or she has been during the course of his or her life is a means of accepting death as an ending to life. When this does not occur, despair and fear of death may prevail. Death then negates the possibility of resolving one's unlived or meaningless life.

Aging prepares us for death. But the reality is that few people have the capability to accomplish this final task, and many people are ill prepared to face their death. In the past, sudden death was feared because the "perfect" death was one that gave the person time to prepare for death. Today, the opposite is true. A sudden death is wished for and the fear of dying rather than the fear of death has gained precedence.

Interventions focused on the elderly who are grieving both physical and symbolic losses begin with the caregiver's awareness of his or her personal beliefs and attitudes about aging. Avoidance or fear of getting old might cause the caregiver to avoid, neglect, or deny important feelings or sensitive decisions surrounding aging losses. If the aging person is a spouse or parent, it is important to look at personal losses that are emerging because of the changing relationship.

Anything the caregiver can do to make the elderly person feel good about him- or herself and maintain his or her self- esteem will add to quality of life. It will be helpful to encourage the person to talk about how he or she feels about getting older and to allow for verbal and appropriate physical expression of the reactions to loss. It may be difficult at times to hear negative reactions, but realize that this is a necessary part of the grieving process and assists in possible changes.

Most likely, the aging person has already been thinking about the changes and losses going on in his or her life. Now might be a good time to begin a life review. In this review, a person remembers and shares events and experiences in an effort to bring some sense or meaning to his or her life. It is important that each of us tells our own unique life story to someone. Solicitation of family members able to listen patiently can be extremely beneficial to the ones who are ready and willing to engage in this process. Just a quiet presence may be enough. Remember, too, that the elderly are not just grieving for aging losses but may also be experiencing multiple losses that have been denied in the past. They may be repeating the details of a loss over and over again because it does not fit into their belief system and seems unexplainable.

If the care recipient is able, encourage communication, activities, and visits with peers and friends. Many cities have support groups for senior citizens that can be an arena for meeting many needs the caregiver will be unable to meet. Participation in church-based groups and activities also may be particularly meaningful.

Dying

I was cutting Dad's hair as he sat up in his hospital bed. Tears began to roll down my face as I realized that this would be the last time I would ever cut his hair. My Daddy was dying. I hoped that he didn't see the tears. We finished and I sat down in front of the bed. Dad had not said much all day. He was withdrawing, moving farther away and leaving us. My brother propped up the pillow behind his head, trying to make him more comfortable. Just then, a nurse came in to check him. She commented on his great haircut. She said, "John, you sure are lucky to have such good kids. They're really taking good care of you." In five seconds this nurse-messenger said what I had been waiting to hear from my father all my life: that I was a good kid. He could never or would never say it but, finally, somebody did. Such a gift could have come only from God. My dad died the next morning.

The anticipatory grief that is felt by the dying person is also felt by the family and the caregiver. The emotional reactions are similar but the dying person may feel his or her grief more intensely. During this time, grief becomes a part of life, and everyone is affected. The major task for the caregiver as the care recipient enters the dying process is to make sure that he or she is surrounded by who and what is important to him or her, and to encourage as much personal autonomy and choice as possible. It is important to help the person identify and verbalize sources of anxiety about dying.

The dying person expects to be treated the same as always, and not all of his emotional reactions are because he is dying. He may be angry because he does not want to do something you want him to do! Open, honest communication is important. It is more acceptable to disagree with the dying person about something, than to placate or condescend. Dying changes relationships and families, so consider how this awareness of death can enhance the remaining time. Also, it is important to avoid treating the dying, emotionally and socially, as if they are not there or are already dead.

People die in different ways, and the dying process is as unique as a person's life. Stress and grief response patterns to the dying experience can be generally acted out as fighting against the possibility of death (conflict, anger, struggle), fleeing (denial, avoidance), or flow (adaptation, acceptance).

In recent years, models of dying and expected emotional responses have helped people come to a better understanding of the dying process. On the other side of the coin, some of these models have created unrealistic expectations about what is supposed to happen in order for a person to die an appropriate death. These expectations can cause undue pain and burden for the dying as well as a high level of frustration and sense of failure for the caregiver and the family.

Not everyone fits into Elisabeth Kubler-Ross' study of young cancer patients. This is particularly true of the dying elderly. Her five psychological stages of dying are denial, anger, bargaining, depression, and acceptance. Although some of these responses may occur, to expect that the dying patient must experience or successfully work through each stage is unrealistic and may satisfy the needs of the grieving person more than those of the dying person. Although encouraging expression is important in caring for the dying, not everyone will want to talk. If the care recipient spoke little through most of his or her life, chances are that he or she will not change now.

Hope of change is another consideration for high expectations. The dying process can catalyze changes in a person's attitudes and behavior, but many people die with no loving or meaningful exchange and with unresolved conflict in their relationships. Some may become more self-centered and withdrawn and lash out at others.

At some point in the process of dying, it may be beneficial to give the dying person permission to let go and relinquish the relationships and life he or she has known. This is difficult for both the care recipient and the caregiver. Timing is of the essence, and it may be necessary to speak to someone else who may know the dying person to ascertain the best course of action. As the dying person lets go of his or her outer life, the focus may become more inward. This is a gradual process that happens naturally in some aging people.

The dying person experiences some of the same grief reactions that the bereaved experiences after another's death. Dealing with grief will include identifying the losses, expressing feelings, and reviewing and finishing unfinished business with relatives and friends. The dying person may experience a loss of self-esteem, due to a debilitating or terminal illness not experienced by the bereaved after a death. Being cognizant of some of the fears the individual is experiencing will be helpful in reassuring the dying elderly that these reactions are normal.

Fear of the unknown, fear of loneliness, and fear of the loss of family and friends are common. There may also be a fear of loss of body parts or of disability. Conveying the necessity of grieving for these losses and reaffirming the person's value beyond the deterioration of the body may alleviate some of this fear. The possibility of regression may be frightening to the patient. If there is regression, this running away and disengagement from life should be accommodated. There should be a reduction in stimulation, and more quiet time should be spent with family and caregiver.

The need to have control—and the fear of losing it—can be a particularly threatening situation for the dying care recipient. It is critical that the caregiver allow as many opportunities for patient control without denying the reality of the dying situation.

Perhaps the most difficult and destructive aspect of death for both the dying patient and the caregiver is physical pain and emotional suffering. Sometimes, even with medication and the lessening of physical pain, no matter what we do or how much we care, we cannot take away the suffering of the ill or dying person. This can cause tremendous emotional suffering for the caregiver. The dying person may suffer if there seems to be no meaning to the pain or if he or she perceives that the pain represents punishment.

The caregiver's role is not necessarily to facilitate peaceful acceptance of death. In fact, this may not be possible, since dying forces one to say goodbye and can be met with struggling and resistance. The caregiver can only be present, listen, and bear the pain with the dying. Minimizing the loss of wholeness, isolation, and rejection for the dying person may be all that can be accomplished.

The caregiver may encourage the dying older person to perform some practical tasks that may assist in preparation for death. If the care recipient is unable to do them, the caregiver can take on the tasks but ask the dying person to assist in decision making. Some of these practical matters can be beneficial in the aging process as a means of addressing the reality that no one lives forever. With acceptance of that reality, there are some things the elderly can take responsibility for, thus lessening the burden on others. Some of the tasks can give the dying care recipient a sense of control during a chaotic time. Arranging for a variety of affairs, such as getting the will in order, settling financial matters, providing for the welfare of others, making funeral arrangements, leaving messages for friends and relatives, although uncomfortable to deal with, can provide relief to everyone involved, if handled sensitively.

Another area in which the dying can exercise control is in the planning and decision making surrounding medical care. Recipient input into choices about doctors, medications, curative versus comforting measures, and location of treatment and death can alleviate some of the stress caregivers feel in having to make these decisions.

Helping the dying elderly live fully and deal with their own grief about losing their world and their self is both physically and emotionally exhausting and stressful. The caregiver is not only mourning the dying person's loss, but also mourning his or her own loss, especially if the dying person is a spouse, parent, or close relative. Losing aspects of the person you are caring for is particularly painful. Because this partial grief cannot come to resolution until after death, a sort of limbo state of existence begins to drain the caregiver.

At this point, these multiple grief experiences can push the caregiver into a bereavement overload. Helping anyone to die is an immense and sacred responsibility and it is important for the caregiver to recognize his or her limitations and capabilities and that help may be needed.

Ask the care recipient's physician about the availability of hospice services for the dying and see about respite services for yourself. In the past, resources for dealing with grief issues were scarce. But the availability of more support groups dealing specifically with grief or loss surrounding certain health concerns such as cancer, diabetes, and Alzheimer's disease are increasing emotional support for both the dying and the caregiver.

If the dying person's or your own grief reactions are overwhelming or become complicated, consider counseling or therapy with a professional who is knowledgeable in the area of grief. Senior citizens' agencies, clergy, and hospices may be a good place to call for information. Remember, it is important that the caregiver be able to ask for and get help. This can free the caregiver to take time to do some of his or her own grief work.

Grief Work

How people deal with their grief from aging, illness, dying, death, and caregiving will ultimately influence the quality of their lives. Grief can be dealt with by passively allowing it to have its way with us, or it can be dealt with by actively engaging in the tasks necessary to bring about true resolution and reconciliation of the responses and reactions to loss. Grief work really is a lot of work!

There are at least five tasks in mourning that will be helpful in resolving grief:

- Accept the reality of the loss—accept what is, not what you would like reality to be.
- Experience the emotional pain of grief. This may mean taking the time to allow the pain to be felt and to nurture oneself in the process.
- Shift the relationship with the deceased person from one of presence to one of memory.
- Develop a new self-identity without the deceased.
- Find a sense of meaning in your loss.

Some of this grief work can be begun during the anticipatory grief period; however, much of the intensity, difficulty, and resolution will remain after death.

There are numerous interventions and steps in grief work that can facilitate the process of grieving. The first step is to develop an awareness of the loss and face reality. Encourage verbalization of feelings by listening and accepting without judgment, allowing for crying, reviewing, and repetition. Do not be afraid to mention your loss or your loved one and do not be afraid to show your feelings, care, or concern. It is comforting to know that one does not have to take the pain away from another or rescue him or her from being human.

When dealing with grief, it is good to acknowledge that most people want to avoid the pain, although all of us ultimately have to go through it. Avoid trying to "fix" anyone or telling them what to do. Most people need to be listened to without comment, and a quiet presence can have a healing effect. Acknowledge your helplessness and admit that you do not know the answers to the mysteries of life and death.

In response to grief reactions allow yourself and others to be wherever they are in their grief. If there is denial, allow it and do not try to "break through" it. Recognize ambivalent feelings, knowing that there are conflicting forces and feelings within all of us. Permitting depression will increase the likelihood that it will be resolved. It is appropriate to wallow, whine, wail, and moan when you are in grief. When else would you express these feelings?

Allow for anger and other uncomfortable emotions. Try to understand why they are so uncomfortable. Screaming, hitting pillows, or kicking paper bags in privacy can do a lot to circumvent internalization of grief.

Try to identify and express needs during the grieving process. If this is something that you are unable to do alone, ask for help. The best asset in grief and caregiving is to have good friends and/or family to count on. Educate yourself and other mourners about grief. Buy or borrow books that will help to understand the particular aspects of grief that you are struggling with. Be your own expert and write about your experiences in a journal. Write a letter to the person you lost or are losing, telling them how you feel. Ask for and give forgiveness for any wrong. Paint or draw a good memory or dream. Join a support group and make a decision to be healthy and whole again.

Some of the most helpful actions in working through grief are the symbols and rituals that give meaning and a sense of connection with the deceased. Families who have experienced meaningful religious services or memorials seem to have an easier time adjusting to their loss. A visible or symbolic reminder of the deceased person is beneficial to the survivors. Perhaps planting a tree or making a donation in their honor will be enough. A special place to visit to be connected to the memory of a person can be a safe and healing way of grieving. At holidays, birthdays, or anniversary days, grief may become especially intense, even after progress has been made toward resolution. Allow some time to grieve on these special occasions.

If there are children in the family, include them in the grief process. Children's grief is sometimes expressed more through behaviors than through talk, but it is imperative to ask children how they are doing. Really listen to their responses and take the time to acknowledge their reactions and feelings. Make children a part of the caregiving and grief process on some level. They will learn a great deal about the grieving process by watching how those around them handle it.

As much care should be given to you, the caregiver, as you are giving or have given to the care recipient. Be gentle with yourself as with anyone who is grieving. Be patient and lower your expectations of yourself. Take a break from grief once in a while. Nurture yourself, get someone to help you get away for a few hours. Remember, you do not have to do it all by yourself.

Everyone has limitations and needs help once in awhile. Beware of addictions. Take a walk regularly, get daily rest and relaxation, get a massage, and give time to your loving and supportive relationships. Do not forget to laugh and play. Remember where you hid your sense of humor.

For those bereaved after a lifetime of involvement with a spouse, parent, or relative, it seems impossible to believe that life will be better again. The truth may be that life will not be better or worse, but it will be different. The loss may unwillingly catapult the survivor into another life, and the best possible grief work will be to remain open in spite of the desire to close oneself off from the possibility of new life.

References

Averill, J.R., and Nunley, E.P. (1988). "Grief as an Emotion and as a Disease: A Social-Constructionist Perspective." *Journal of Social Issues*, 44, 79–95.

Bass, D.M., L.S. Noelker, A.L. Townsend, and G.T. Deimling, (1990). "Losing an Aged Relative: Perceptual Differences between Spouse and Adult Children." *Omega*, 21, 22–40.

Eakes, G.G. (1985). "The Relationship between Death Anxiety and Attitudes toward the Elderly among Nursing Staff." *Death Studies*, 9, 163–172.

Fulton, R. (1987). "The Many Faces of Grief." *Death Studies*, 11, 243–256.

Fulton, R. and G. Owen (1988). "Death and Society in Twentieth Century America." *Omega*, 18, 379-395.

Goebel, B.L. and B.E. Boeck (1987). "Ego Integrity and Fear of Death: A Comparison of Institutionalized and Independently Living Older Adults." *Death Studies*, 11, 193–204.

Gray, R.E. (1988). "Meaning of Death: Implications for Bereavement Theory." *Death Studies*, 12, 309–317.

Huber, R. and J.W. Gibson (1990). "New Evidence for Anticipatory Grief." *Hospice Journal*, 6, 49–67.

Kubler-Ross, E. *On Death and Dying*. New York: Macmillan, 1969.

Lannie, V.J. (1984). "The Positive Aspects of Anguish." American *Journal of Hospice Care*, 33–35.

Mailik, M.D. (1983). "Understanding Illness and Aging." *Gerontological Social Work*, 113–126.

Malkinson, R. (1987). "Helping the Being Helped: The Support Paradox." *Death Studies*, 11, 205–219.

Parkes, C.M. (1987). "Models of Bereavement Care." *Death Studies*, 11, 257–261.

Parkes, C.M. (1988). "Research: Bereavement." *Omega*, 18, 365-377.

Parkes, C.M. (1988). "Bereavement as a Psychosocial Transition: Processes of Adaptation to Change." *Journal of Social Issues*, 44, 53–65.

Rabins, P.V. (1984). "Management of Dementia in the Family Context." *Psychosomatics*, 25, 369-375.

Rando, T.A. *Grief, Dying and Death: Clinical Interventions for Caregivers*. Champaign, IL: Research Press, 1984.

Rando, T.A., ed. *Loss and Anticipatory Grief*. Lexington, MA, Lexington Books, 1986.

Rando, T.A. Grieving: *How to Go on Living When Someone You Love Dies*. Lexington, MA, Lexington Books, 1988.

Reed, P.G. (1986). "Death Perspectives and Temporal Variables in Terminally Ill and Healthy Adults." *Death Studies*, 10, 467–478.

Retsinas, J. (1988). "A Theoretical Reassessment of the Applicability of Kubler-Ross's Stages of Dying." *Death Studies*, 12, 207–216.

Robinson, P.J. and F. Fleming, (1984). "Differentiating Grief and Depression." *Hospice Journal*, 3, 77–78.

Rosenblatt, P.C. (1988). "Grief: The Social Context of Private Feelings." *Journal of Social Issues*, 44, 67–78.

Roy, R. (1986). "A Psychosocial Perspective on Chronic Pain and Depression in the Elderly." *Social Work in Health Care*, 12, 27–36.

Sanders, C.M. (1982). "Effects of Sudden vs. Chronic Illness Death on Bereavement Outcome." *Omega*, 13, 227–241.

Schmall, V.L. and C.C. Pratt, (1989). "Family Caregiving and Aging, Strategies for Support." Aging and Family Therapy, 71–87.

Stephenson, J.S. and D. Murphy, (1986). "Existential Grief; The Special Case of the Chronically Ill and Disabled." *Death Studies*, 10, 135–145.

Viney, L.L, Y.N. Benjamin, and C. Preston, (1989). "Mourning and Reminiscence: Parallel Psychotherapeutic Processes for Elderly People." *International Journal Aging and Human Development*, 28, 239–249.

Viorst, J. *Necessary Losses*. New York: Simon & Schuster, 1986.

Wasow, M. (1984). "Get Out of My Potato Patch: A Biased View of Death and Dying." *Health and Social Work*, 261–267.

Weinberg, N. (1985). "The Health Care Social Worker's Role in Facilitating Grief Work: An Empirical Study." *Social Work in Health Care*, 10, 107–117.

Williams, F.R. (1989). "Bereavement and the Elderly: The Role of the Psychotherapist." *Aging and Family Therapy*, 225–241.

Wolfelt, A.D. (1987). "Understanding Common Patterns of Avoiding Grief." *Thanatos*, 12, 2–5.

Worden, J.W. *Grief Counseling and Grief Therapy.* New York:Springer, 1982.

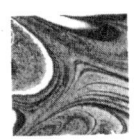

Profile

"Yolanda" is a 76-year-old woman who provided care for her husband, "Eligio," for seven and a half years. At the beginning of her caregiving experience, Yolanda did not understand the prognosis of the illness that was affecting her husband. Neither did she realize that the emotional, financial and physical difficulties she was experiencing were just the beginning of a more demanding and complex situation. One thing was clear since the beginning of the illness: Eligio was not going to a nursing home regardless of how much physical, emotional and financial burden his illness would bring to the family.

As was customary in the Cuban culture, a culture very much alive among elderly Cubans, Yolanda married Eligio for better or for worse, until death do them part. She would take care of him at the expense of her own health. Yolanda never thought that her new responsibility as a caregiver was any different than her responsibility as a wife. Therefore, having options as to what to do in her caregiver role was unimaginable. In her world, being a wife is being a caregiver. Her perception is supported by the fact that in the Hispanic culture, the word *caregiver* does not exist. In 1984, at the time of the onset of his renal failure, Eligio was convinced he would be able to resume his normal life after a couple of dialysis treatments. He never realized that the dialysis treatments would become a permanent part of his life. By his third year of treatment, Eligio had gone through three operations for a shunt and suffered two strokes and the complications of an ulcer. His initial optimism began to wear off, and his physical stamina began to fail. It was at this time that the family was first exposed to the concept of a living will, and even though it was not in total agreement with their Catholic upbringing, every member of the family, including Eligio, prepared one. This was a crucial event in their lives because, at the time Eligio signed his living will, he was in full control of his faculties. By doing that, he relieved his wife and daughter of any future guilt related to his death.

Eligio, the physically strong and powerful person, became confined to a wheel chair, began to have problems with his memory and experienced extreme personality changes. While the attention of the family was concentrated on Eligio's physical and mental deterioration, his wife of 40 years quietly abandoned her life and began assuming responsibility for keeping him alive regardless of the cost. The three-times-a-week visit to the dialysis treatment facility became her only social gathering. His constant hospitalizations became her only outings. His physical therapy rehabilitation program became her only distraction. Yolanda's interest in her grandchildren became secondary to her obsession with keeping Eligio clean, well fed and alive.

For two years prior to his death, Eligio was bedridden, and moving him from the bed to the wheel chair to go to dialysis treatment became a physical challenge for Yolanda. Eligio died last year, and Yolando feels that all her sacrifices were worth it because she had fulfilled the cultural expectations of her generation. She was there until the end.

From a cultural perspective, Yolanda was doing what was expected of her. Her value system gave her enough rewards to keep her going, even at times when it required a superhuman effort. Yolanda found happiness and comfort in the fact that she provided love and care at home for her husband.

Their daughter's advice to those in similar situations:

- Cultural values play a key role in defining burden and in relieving the caregiver of his or her guilt. In seeking help for the caregiver, attempt to find persons or organizations that will be sensitive to the caregiver's belief system.
- Fulfilling cultural expectations may be as important to some as obtaining physical respite. While the temptation may be strong to intervene, friends and family members may find that they serve the caregiver best simply by being there as a source of comfort and emotional support.
- A care recipient needs to define what he or she considers to be quality of life prior to the onset of dementia. Preparing a living will is a good way to do it.

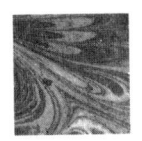

Introduction to Financial Planning

Caregivers are expected to always be in good humor, to be experts in psychology and medicine, and to manage their loved one's business affairs as efficiently and expertly as Lee Iacocca managed the Chrysler Corporation. In many families, the caregiver will encounter coaching from an endless stream of Monday morning quarterbacks.

For some caregivers, the best decision may be to hire a trustworthy advisor to manage their loved one's financial affairs. But, as in any business dealing, choose your advisor carefully. The best choice may be an attorney, accountant, bank trust officer, financial planner, or a combination of professionals. Regardless of who is selected, that person should be:

- licensed in Florida
- have experience specific to your requirements
- be able to answer your questions so that you completely understand any advice or recommendation they offer
- be willing to clarify fees and be able to establish them at the outset of the relationship
- follow the standards for risk you outline
- have integrity and be discreet
- be willing, if necessary, to work with other professionals involved in caring for your loved one.

Quick tips

DEVELOP A COMPREHENSIVE FINANCIAL PLAN.

The best statement on planning was probably made by Dwight D. Eisenhower: "Plans are nothing, planning is everything."

Planning is an opportunity to think through a situation and select the best course of action. If the situation changes perhaps the plan will also change, but the process of planning helps avoid surprises and assures that alternatives have been considered.

MAKE WELL-INFORMED DECISIONS.

Making good decisions requires that adequate information is available for review prior to the time the decision is needed—that the decision is made prior to the time when taking no action is the same as having made a decision. One way to be able to make well considered decisions is to have in place a process for deciding. This process includes:

- following the criteria set in the financial plan
- gathering enough information to be able to consider each plausible course of action
- comparing the pros and cons of each course of action with the criteria previously established and making a choice
- getting advice on the choice
- acting on your decision
- following up on the decision to see that your instructions were carried out accurately and completely and that the results were what you intended.

NEVER INTERMINGLE THE CARE RECIPIENT'S FINANCES WITH YOUR OWN.

Doing so can only lead to guilt and self-doubt, accusations of impropriety from family members, a visit from the Internal Revenue Service, or all three. While this may seem unnecessary, especially if you and the care recipient live in the same house, it is important and may be necessary to show that your loved one is eligible for financial, medical, or social assistance.

Keeping separate financial arrangements can be accomplished by:

- having separate checking and savings accounts
- keeping separate records of transactions including purchases and bill paying
- providing receipts when money or services are exchanged
- having an impartial third-party such as an accountant or bank officer review your records.

KEEP A JOURNAL THAT DOCUMENTS YOUR ACTIONS.

This is especially important if your loved one is unable to make financial decisions without your assistance or intervention.

The journal should include:

- the time and date of the action
- the amount of the transactions
- your rationale for initiating the action.

Caregivers Handbook

PREPARE MONTHLY OR QUARTERLY REPORTS, REGARDLESS OF YOUR LOVED ONE'S MENTAL CONDITION OR FINANCIAL STATUS.

If he or she is able to do so, have him or her initial each page of the report in ink. Otherwise, arrange for an attorney, accountant, or guardian to review the report and initial it. If there is no one else to review the document, mail a copy to yourself in a sealed envelope date-stamped by the post office. Keep the unopened record on file.

IF AN INVESTMENT OR PURCHASE SOUNDS TOO GOOD TO BE TRUE, IT PROBABLY IS TOO GOOD TO BE TRUE.

The most important step in deciding what investments you will make is to develop an investment guideline that allocates assets according to your particular goals, needs, and tolerance for risk, considering the care recipient's age, expenses, and medical needs.

10

Financial Planning

C. Colburn Hardy

For lack of planning, security is lost; for lack of security, dignity is lost; for lack of dignity, the man is lost.
—Tony Lamb

Much of what concerns an elderly person and his/her caregiver revolves around how to manage money and other assets to pay for daily living expenses and for the additional costs—especially those of health care. Even with careful financial planning and investment management, there will be concern over unanticipated expenses and the senior's inability to continue to manage his/her own affairs. This is the time when a caregiver and advisers can be important. Wise planning and implementation can assure greater income for a longer period and maintain assets for a life—a very important factor with more people living longer and the persistent erosion of inflation.

Each situation is unique: many are complicated and all are difficult because so many older people are reluctant to give up control of their finances. At some point, the role of the caretaker and advisers can be essential in helping to provide ample income and to maintain assets as long as possible, hopefully for life. This chapter outlines proven effective methods of investing, spells out *DOs* and *DON'Ts,* and shows the steps to take—and to avoid—to assure a financially secure environment.

Getting Started

To understand financial responsibilities and to make the most rewarding, most comforting and most beneficial use of resources, it is essential to know the individual's worth—assets minus liabilities—and current anticipated income.

STEPS TO TAKE

- Itemize current and projected income: Social Security, pensions, investments, and possible inheritances
- Inventory all assets in two categories, *fixed*: (home, land, furniture, property, collectibles, automobiles, boats, and electrical/electronic equipment) and *flexible*: (bank accounts, securities, real estate, pension plans, annuities, life insurance, and debts payable to the individual)
- List all liabilities: mortgage, loans payable to another, bills, credit card balances, charge accounts, and charitable pledges.

From these bases, rough out a budget for expenditures for the current year and, after several months of proving out, project these costs taking into account inflation.

Calculating Income

When possible, reinvest all income from investments—interest, dividends, and realized capital gains. This will compound returns by earning income on income: in five years, with an 8 percent annual rate of return, capital will grow by 147 percent; in 10 years, with a 10 percent annual yield, it will grow by 259 percent.

Find out where the senior stands, financially, today, and where he or she can be expected to be in the foreseeable future, at intervals of no more than five years.

Financial Planning

The one sure source of income in retirement is Social Security, the governmental program that requires tax deductions while working and cash benefits after work. Often, this is supplemented by pensions—from the employer and by individual savings.

SOCIAL SECURITY

Social Security checks will be an important source of income for all retirees so, to be sure that proper benefits will be received, call your local Social Security office or (800) 772-1213 and ask for a Personal Earnings and Benefit Estimate Statement (PEBES). For identification, state the name, date of birth, current address, and phone number of the beneficiary.

The PEBES will list: (1) earning history; (2) how much has been paid into the individual's account; (3) current benefits or, if not yet eligible, an estimate of future checks at retirement, for disability and survivors. There's no charge if the information is to be sent to the beneficiary or to the person requesting the information in his or her behalf. There is up to a $5 charge for information sent elsewhere.

Retirement benefits can start at age 62, at a rate of 20 percent less than those that will be paid when the beneficiary reaches age 65. This will change to age 67 early in the next century. In 1993, the average annual Social Security payment at age 65 is $9,828, with an additional 50 percent added when a non-working spouse is involved. Currently there is a Federal income tax for beneficiaries with income over $25,000 (for singles) or $32,000 (for joint filers). It appears likely that these limits will be lowered in the future.

If your loved one is unable to manage his or her financial affairs, the checks will be sent to the responsible individual or agency and the money used solely for the use or care of the beneficiary. It will not be used to pay past debts.

Beware of Rip-Offs:

By mail and, sometimes, in person, hustlers will try to exploit fears of retirees as to the future of Social Security benefits. The "warning" comes in an official-looking envelope with "Social Security" emblazoned on the outside and, within, a dire headline that retirement benefits are being threatened by new taxes, diversion of funds, and the possibility that Congress will fail to approve an annual COLA (Cost of Living Adjustment). It may include a dramatic plea for funds to help oppose such actions.

Do not send money to these individuals or organizations. The only person your contribution will benefit is the perpetrator of the rip-off.

CHOOSING ADVISERS

Even when the assets of the senior are modest, it is wise to choose advisers such as a lawyer, accountant, broker, and financial consultant. Hopefully, these will become long-term relationships that will involve personalities as well as performance. Look for individuals who have had experience with similar situations, are readily available, charge reasonable fees, and know how to relate to older folks. Empathy and trust are essential for decisions to be made promptly and amicably. *Do not hesitate to make changes when you are persuaded that they will be in the best interest of the care recipient.*

In most cases, it will be wise to continue to work with the same individuals or firms that you or the care recipient have consulted in the past but, first, review each choice in terms of future requirements and financial resources. Like all other service providers, financial advisers have to be paid.

In the event that you are starting with a clean slate, you should identify potential advisors by asking friends and local business acquaintances. They should be licensed to practice or do business in Florida and have specific experience in areas of need. They also should:

- clearly spell out costs and the sources of all fees or commissions;
- provide written guidelines for decisions;
- express willingness to work with other professionals
- make available written and verbal recommendations as to the integrity and ability of themselves and their firms.

MAKING THE MOST OF ASSETS

Now that you know the available assets and projected expenses, let's discuss some of the productive steps to take with investments to provide the most rewarding, most lasting financial returns: basically, to assure the maximum, safe income for the longest period of time.

This is the time to plan carefully, to set strict rules, and to be very conservative. Too often, after the death of one partner, when the estate is, or appears to be substantial, the survivor will be overwhelmed by this "wealth" and will be determined to enjoy the rest of his or her life: new clothes, furniture, car, entertainment, and travel. Such largess can be temporarily exciting but devastating over the long-term. Even when there is only one survivor, costs will rise, for health care, assisted living, home repairs and replacement, and the like.

This caveat is especially pertinent when personal pension plans, such as IRAs, are involved. Under IRS rules, withdrawals must start no later than age 70.5 and be completed while both partners are "actuarialy alive" (i.e., when both husband and wife are age 70, a time span of 18.3 years).

At this age, there still will be: (1) checks from Social Security, though, probably with smaller annual COLAS; (2) benefits from employer-sponsored pension plans which, usually, are paid for life; and (3) income from savings investments.

HOW LONG WILL SAVINGS LAST?

To project how long savings/investments will last in retirement, at various rates of return and withdrawal, use this table:

Annual withdrawals	\multicolumn{4}{c}{Growth rate}	
	6%	7%	10%	12%
10%	15	20		
12%	11	14	18	
15%	8	9	11	14

(Years)

Thus, if the investments total $100,000 and are invested at an average annual yield of 10 percent ($10,000 income in Year 1), you can withdraw 12 percent for 18 years before exhausting the total.

Annuities

A convenient way to assure income for life is an annuity. These are policies, sold by insurance companies, that guarantee payment to the retiree and/or beneficiary of a monthly sum for life, starting at a pre-set age, often age 65 or 70. They are widely used to supplement or replace pension benefits. But they involve some risks: if the senior dies soon after the payments start, the costs will be high. But if he or she lives long, the returns will be very rewarding.

Annuities can be purchased at any age, with a single sum or by periodic savings. The premium is a non-tax-deductible expense. The income, from interest, dividends, and appreciation is tax-deferred until withdrawn. At that time, the gains are taxed as ordinary income with the balance tax-free as a return of capital.

Example: $10,000 investment; 9 percent rate of return, payout over 20 years (before fees and/or taxes)*

Years Accumulated	Annuity Value	Payout
5	$12,620	$1,049
10	16,295	1,396
15	21,449	1,883
20	28,678	2,565

Annual maintenance cost: 2% plus $30; beneficiary in 32% tax bracket.

An increasingly popular type of annuity is the Pooled Income Plan (PIP). This combines philanthropy, a tax benefit and lifetime income. The donor receives an immediate tax deduction based on a formula based on the value of a gift plus lifetime income for self and spouse. If, for example, Horatio, age 80, needs extra income and wants to help his college, he might donate 300 shares of K-Mart, worth $11,925. He bought the stock at $12/share, so he has an $8,325 capital gain which, if he sold the stock, would trigger a tax of almost $2,200.

In this scenario, Horatio gets a tax deduction of $4,464 and can count on annual income of about $960 as long as he and/or his spouse live. When both he and his spouse die, the shares become the property of the university.

Investing

With all investments—personal, pension plan or trust fund—insist on quality. Corporations, governments, and agencies should be rated *A* or higher by Standard & Poor's or Moody's Investors Service, available from a broker or banker or the public library).

This means:

- with *bonds*, issuers with ample cash, income more than sufficient to pay interest, amortization and redemption; securities whose prices are quoted in the financial press and readily available from brokers. *Invest backward: determine when the money will be needed and buy bonds due to mature at that time.*
- with *stocks*, familiar corporations whose goods or services you recognize, are widely used and have proven to be successful over time.

Specifically, here are criteria used for investment by one major, successful professional money manager: invest only in shares traded on an American stock exchange, in companies that have capital and surplus of at least $40 million, that for the past 10 years have earned a minimum of 11 percent on equity capital (stockholders' money) and that have boosted profits by at least 6 percent annually, preferably 15 percent.

For *income*: shares of utilities and banks that pay ever-higher dividends of 4 percent to 6 percent and continue to boost profits so that the values of their stocks rise to achieve total average annual returns of 10 percent to 12 percent.

For *growth*: stocks of financially strong, profitable companies that have fairly consistent records of higher profits with a profit rate of at least 15 percent annually.

CERTIFICATES OF DEPOSIT (CDS)

CDs are issued by banks or savings and loan associations, usually in units of $1,000 with maturities of from three months to five years. Currently, yields are a low 3 percent to 5 percent but, in periods of high interest, they can be more rewarding, safe, and convenient.

BANK ACCOUNTS

Bank accounts usually are for check-writing but also pay modest interest. These are no longer needed for emergencies, as a credit card can be used to purchase airline tickets and obtain cash.

MONEY MARKET FUNDS

Available from financial institutions and brokers, these are pooled investments that pay, and compound, interest daily. They are handy, liquid, and often used with brokerage accounts to hold temporary receipts while waiting for new investment opportunities.

TREASURY BILLS

Treasury bills are short-term issues with maturities of 90 days, 180 days, and one year. The minimum holding is $10,000, with the purchase price reflecting the interest to maturity; i.e. a 360-day, 6 percent bill, costs $9,400 and, a year later, can be cashed in for $10,000.

TREASURY NOTES

These may be purchased in units of $1,000 with a minimum purchase of $5,000. They mature in one to 10 years. Yields are competitive.

TREASURY BONDS

These bonds have a $5,000 face value with maturities up to 30 years. They offer high yields and are not callable, meaning that you can select a redemption date to fit your future financial needs.

Treasury issues can be purchased at any financial institution. The interest is taxable on federal, but not on state or local tax returns.

ZERO COUPON BONDS

"Zeros" are an excellent investment for a pension plan or trust account, but are seldom suitable for personal portfolios. These debt issues are sold at prices far below face value: 20-year, $1,000 bonds sell at $225, for an annual yield of 7 percent.

Zeros pay no interest but, each year, their value rises by the amount of the imputed interest. This appreciation is tax-deferred with fiduciary funds but is taxable to the individual even though no interest is received. When you do invest in zeros, choose the maturity date at a time when the proceeds will be needed.

U.S. SAVINGS BONDS

Savings bonds are 100 percent safe, and provide welcome yields: for EE Savings Bonds, available at half price ($12.50 for a $25 face value) with issues up to $10,000 each. When held for five years, they pay the higher of 6 percent or 85 percent of average yield of five-year treasury bonds. The interest is not subject to state or local income tax or to federal tax at redemption. They can be rolled over, tax-free, into HH savings bonds which pay 6 percent taxable interest for 20 years.

MORTGAGE PASS-THROUGHS

These are loans on homes and apartments that are packaged and sold, usually in units of $25,000. The interest, amortization, and repayments are passed-through to investors monthly and, when there is refinancing or repayment, a portion of those dollars also is paid. The yields are high, currently up to 8 percent.

Most of the original mortgages have been for 30 years but, with lower interest rates, repayments and refinancing have been frequent. The average life of a pool of Government National Mortgage Association

(Ginnie Mae) Pass Throughs is now about 12 years, not a long-term investment for bonds.

For most investors, the best choice will be shares of mutual funds that can be purchased for as little as $1,000. They continue for many years as the income can be reinvested for compounding. Similarly safe debt investments are available from other federal agencies.

Collateralized Mortgage Obligations (CMOs) are similar debt packages available from financial institutions. The yields are higher but there are no guarantees or insurance.

Key investments to the individual

With all types of securities, determine the individual's (and spouse's) tolerance for risk. This is essential with bonds as their prices move opposite to the cost of money: *up* when interest rates drop; *down* when they rise. With stocks, prices will reflect corporate profitability, over time.

- Invest for a specific goal: for income when there is a need for a steady flow of dividends or interest; for growth when it is possible to wait for a year or two for worthwhile appreciation.
- Diversify: no more than 20% of a portfolio in any one company—except for U.S. Government debt.
- Beware of hot tips: "sure to rise" stocks or overly high-yielding bonds.
- Never invest in anything that you do not understand, such as special types of securities or "can't miss opportunities". If they sound too good to be true, they probably are.
- Watch out for scams: special "investments" that cost less and/or pay more than standard opportunities. Be doubly cautious when the offer involves church groups, health care agencies, special tax breaks or "little-known quirks in the law."

MUNICIPAL BOND INVESTMENT

Always double-check the real returns.

To avoid paying extra income taxes on the interest, many seniors invest in municipal bonds: debt obligations of local, county, and state governments/agencies. When the issuer is head-quartered in their home state, there are no taxes on that income. Such investments are not wise for Florida residents because there is no state income taxes. But they do make sense in high-tax areas of the country.

Be wary of "special opportunities" involving swapping tax-exempt securities. These are highly speculative and, while they may work well sometimes, the risks are high.

COMMON STOCKS FOR TOTAL RETURNS

For fair values, look for stocks that are selling at around 15 times a company's last 12 months earnings: i.e., stocks at $30/share when per share profits are $2.

- Set targets: 25 percent to 33 percent above the price in the next 24 to 30 months (longer in flat/down markets). Thus, if the stock is acquired at $30/share, the target price range should be $38 to $40. When the stock reaches this goal, review the prospects and consider selling.
- Be patient: if the company falters, do not panic when management has a record of profitable performance and authoritative research indicates the probability of a comeback.
- Be quick to sell: if there is any indication of mismanagement or lack of integrity by officers or directors or unfavorable external/political developments. *For all retirees, safety of capital is paramount.*

At all times, the investments should be prudent, as defined, in a still-valid 1830 legal decision:

"All that can be required of a trustee in investing is that he shall conduct himself faithfully and exercise a sound discretion. He is to observe how men of prudence, discretion and intelligence manage their affairs, considering the probable income, as well as the probable safety, of the capital to be invested."

To the degree possible, financial decisions should be made by the care recipient with the assistance of the caregiver and advisers. When he or she no longer is able to do the research and make essential decisions, the assets should be managed according to an overall plan and within pre-determined parameters.

The two goals in counseling and in the financial management of the care recipient's finances should be: (1) safety: maintenance of principal as long and as fully as possible; (2) income to achieve the most rewarding returns"

Choosing Mutual Fund Investments

Unless the care recipient and the caretaker have had experience with investments, the best choice will be to buy shares of mutual funds. These are money management firms that sell shares to investors and use the proceeds to buy securities to meet specific goals: income, growth, balance, or, with special types, tax benefits.

There are two types of mutual funds:

- *Load*: shares are sold through brokers, dealers, and special representatives for commissions of from 8.5 percent for small purchases down to 2 percent for larger, contractual commitments. This fee is deducted from the investment, so less money goes to work: with an 8.5 percent load, $91.50 of every $100. The salesperson handles all details.
- *No-load*: shares are bought directly from the sponsoring firm—by phone or by mail—without commissions. All of the savings are invested, but the investor/representative must do the work: setting up the account, making out checks, and arranging for income to be reinvested or paid out.

With almost all mutual funds, there are charges. A management fee might run 0.5 percent to 2 percent of new assets; "back-end" loads of 4 percent to 6 percent; charges of up to 1.25 percent for reinvestment of income; and, often, special fees for reports and marketing.

KNOW WHAT YOUR OPTIONS ARE

Before making a selection of a management firm and a specific mutual fund, do your homework. Check your public library for reports of the performance for the past five years and annual summaries, such as those in the August issue of *Forbes*, which annually rates funds in both "up" and "down" markets.

Debt Funds

For income, there are mutual funds that invest in debt instruments, such as bonds, preferred stocks, mortgages, and packages of loans. For both taxable and municipal debt, there are two formats:

- *unit trusts*: investments in a basket of debt securities with no change until, as the result of calls, redemptions, and, occasionally, defaults,

the assets drop to about 20 percent of the initial offering. At this point, the fund is closed out and assets distributed to shareholders. The original yield is maintained, and there's only one sales charge. The management fees are small, but for safety's sake, it's best when the unit trust is sponsored by a familiar, reputable organization.
- *managed funds*: where the professionals trade in anticipation of shift in interest rates. If they guess right, the fund will outperform the bond market. If they make mistakes, there can be losses. Be wary.

Keep in mind that changes can be made easily and, often, without extra levies. If the economic outlook shifts or new goals are wise, the investor can switch, usually at no cost, to shares of another fund under the same management but better suited to the new objectives.

BENEFITS OF MUTUAL FUND INVESTMENTS

Once you have selected a fund with objectives that fit your needs, you can expect specific benefits from these pooled investments:

- convenience
- professional management
- lower investment costs than personal control
- automatic compounding of income/realized capital appreciation
- the privilege of exchange for shares of other funds when objective shift
- detailed record-keeping, especially valuable for tax returns
- ability to withdraw cash in specific sums or periodically
- ease of estate settlement.

When Extra Income Is Needed

When expenses continue to outpace income, it's time to consider making greater use of non-productive assets. You might consider a *reverse annuity mortgage* (RAM) in which the homeowner is paid by a savings and loan association or bank a monthly sum based on the current value of her or his home. Repayment is made when the house is sold, usually at death.

Example: Wanda, a 72-year-old widow, owns a $100,000 house free and clear. She receives Social Security and a modest pension, but to be comfortable, she needs an extra $4,000 annual income.

At her local bank, Wanda arranges for a RAM to pay her $350 a month for life, at an interest rate of 9 percent. The loan is insured by the Federal Housing Administration. The income is not taxable.

A RAM can be an excellent source of supplementary income for cash-poor/house rich retirees but: (1) look for an experienced lender as closing costs can run as high as 5 percent of the total loan and (2) ask about adding a line of credit for emergency expenses.

Another option is *refinancing* an existing mortgage to take advantage of the equity in the home, especially when the original loan was at a high rate of interest. Carefully check all costs and benefits because once this decision has been made, there may be little left for heirs. To determine the wisdom—and costs—use this table:

Refinancing cost as a % of new mortgage

		2%	3%	4%
Interest	1%	3 3/4 years	7 years	9+ years
decreases	2%	1 3/4 years	3 years	4 1/2 years

Years to recoup costs

If expenses continue to outpace income, it's time to bridge the gap by making better use of available assets. Steps to consider:

- Cashing in life insurance policies, keeping only enough for death expenses. This can trigger taxes on the difference between the policy cost and current value.
- Selling non-productive assets, such as collections of stamps, coins and art, unused furniture, dishes and tableware, books, and old clothing, to a dealer when they are valuable or at a garage sale for pin money.
- Reducing expenses by canceling magazine subscriptions, dropping memberships in clubs and organizations, eating fewer meals out, taking advantage of bargains such as senior air tickets and off-season travel, and making greater use of no- or low-cost community services.

Financial planning checklist

- Keep client accounts separate and in detail.
- Open a bank account in the name of the care recipient using power of attorney as needed.
- Set up record-keeping files, including:
    (1) a ledger with dates, names, times, and terms of all orders, purchases, commitments
    (2) a folder for bills, statements, and payments
    (3) a separate file for warranties and guarantees.
- Keep a record of all forms, reports, statements, and canceled checks involving tax returns, income, and property.
- Every six months, have an impartial, third-party, preferably a banker, accountant, or lawyer, review all records to make certain income was recorded and payments made and that all accounts balance.
- To protect your position, when substantial sums, responsibilities, relatives, or legal interpretations are involved, keep a "decision journal" to list the time, date, and data on financial actions in which you are involved.

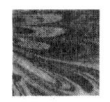

Profile

*A*t age 32, "Connie" has for four years been the primary caregiver or care manager for her 90-year-old grandmother, "Irma." Both Connie and her husband, "Tony," work full time. They have two daughters, aged 2 1/2 and 9 months. Sharing in Irma's care is Connie's 28-year-old married sister, "Kate."

"I grew up believing that you take care of your family," Connie said. "I take care of my grandmother since my biological father can't."

She explained that her father has struggled with alcoholism for many years. His marriage to Connie's and Kate's mother ended in divorce. Then came a string of failed businesses. An only child, he neglected his mother's needs as she grew older, mismanaging and diminishing her financial resources. There has been no communication with him for two years.

During Irma's middle-adult years, she lived an active, independent life, had many friends, and owned and managed an apartment house. In her seventies she had a stroke, but recovered. At age 86, however, Connie and Kate found her living in undesirable conditions with a sitter who left much to be desired and without regular medical care. She was in need of cataract surgery. Most of her friends had died or moved away.

Connie and Kate packed up Irma's things and moved her to Connie's house, 250 miles away. She lived there for six months, until space became available at a local residential center for semi-independent living.

In October 1988, Irma fell and fractured her hip and did not call for help, although an emergency call system was accessible in her room. The fall occurred as the result of a fainting spell due to a previously undiagnosed heart condition. The condition was subsequently corrected with a pacemaker.

Therapy for the fractured hip was unsuccessful, due in part to Irma's depression. After three weeks in a rehabilitation facility, Irma was moved to a nursing home. Connie could not provide nursing care at her home, as her first child had been born only weeks earlier.

Anticipating a future need for nursing home care, Connie had earlier applied for Medicaid and Supplemental Security Income for Irma. The process took two years. Connie found most procedures for gaining access to social services slow and complex, despite the fact that she is employed in the aging services system and generally knows where to go for what.

Both Connie and Kate say they believe that it is important to focus on the care recipient's quality of life. When a loved one is placed in a nursing home, this translates into daily visits, watching as meals are served, observing problems in daily care or in roommate relations, and resisting the use of restraints or a soft diet in place of a regular diet. They also suggest attending monthly family council meetings.

Irma's two young great-granddaughters visit her each weekend. Special treats or snacks add spice to Irma's life, Connie said. The same is true of the new remote control television and motorized bed, recently donated by a relative. Having a daily newspaper delivered is important to Irma, as reading has always been a pleasant part of her morning routine. Without vigilance on the part of the caregiver, "a nursing home can be ghastly," Connie said.

Connie acknowledges that it is not easy to juggle the needs and demands of a husband, children, job, and her grandmother's care. "It's a balancing act," she said. "It's compromises, based on what we believe in." Even though most observers are amazed by her devotion to Irma, Connie sometimes feels guilty.

Her advice to those in similar situations:

- Don't place a person in a nursing home without first exploring other alternatives.
- Regular visits by the caregiver and other family members are essential if the care recipient is placed in a nursing home.
- Involve the care recipient in planning for the future. Provide him or her with frequent assurances that he or she is not being abandoned. Be positive and reassuring. Deal with the care recipient directly and honestly.
- Acknowledge the care recipient's feelings. Never deny them.

- Let the care recipient know what your limitations are.

Connie and her husband share the same beliefs and values. They are already facing the prospect of new caregiving responsibilities.

Tony's father is no longer in good health. Although Tony's parents live 60 miles away, Tony and Connie have bought the house next door to them and moved them into it while the younger couple spends weekends renovating his parents' old house. They are thinking ahead to the future when it can be used for rental income and their own garage can be converted into a "mother-in-*l*aw suite."

As for Connie's relationship with her grandmother, Connie feels that it has changed considerably since she assumed a care management role. Before, they related on a superficial level. Now, they deal with reality and the nitty-gritty details of daily living. Just as Connie was once dependent on her mother, her grandmother is now dependent on her.

The Nursing Home Decision

Pamela Cody

Making the decision to seek nursing home care is an emotional process. In the minds of many older persons, the move to a nursing home marks the time when he or she publicly surrenders independence. Many caregivers view nursing home placement as a sign that they have somehow failed or abandoned their loved ones. The transition from life at home to life in a nursing home is challenging for everyone involved. Living in a nursing home can mean a loss of certain life styles and the things that define a person as an individual: one's own home, personal possessions, and, especially, daily routines. But the right nursing home decision can bring the peace of mind that comes with the knowledge that a loved one is in a safe and loving environment.

There are a variety of circumstances in life that may lead to nursing home placement. A number of people may be involved in making this decision: the prospective resident, family members, friends, clergy, doctors, or social workers. Too often, placement is made without adequate understanding of the needs of the older person. Even the closest families can be torn apart by guilt and fear of the unknown.

The following questions should be considered, taking into account the financial and medical circumstances of the care recipient *and the caregiver*:

- Can the care recipient continue to live independently?
- Does he or she need 24-hour care and supervision?
- Is the care recipient chronically ill, but not sick enough to require the intensive services of a hospital?

- Does he or she need help with daily living activities, such as bathing, dressing, using the toilet, or walking?
- If the care recipient is no longer capable of independent living, is there a friend or family member who is both willing and able to make a lifetime commitment to provide loving care?

Many people who consider nursing home placement have the luxury of time and the availability of a number of nursing homes to choose from. But for others, the need for placement is immediate and the options are few. This leaves little opportunity for planning and selection.

By knowing in advance what to look for in a nursing home, families can feel comfortable in the knowledge that the best possible decision has been made regarding the future of their loved ones.

Chapter 14 includes a section on nursing home placement that lists state contacts that may be of assistance when you feel the time has come to consider this option.

Assuming that there are available beds in your community in your payor category (Medicaid, Medicare or private pay), the first step in selecting a nursing home is to pay a visit to as many area facilities as possible. A complete listing of nursing homes, including information on licensure status, Medicare or Medicaid certification, and number of beds, is available from the Florida Agency for Health Care Administration (AHCA) (see Chapter 14). Set up an appointment with the nursing home administrator or admissions coordinator at each home you plan to visit and have a list of questions ready to ask. The individual you are meeting with should be able to answer all of your questions.

During the initial or subsequent visits, the nursing home representative will ask you for information on your loved one's condition and attempt to determine family expectations of the nursing home. Be prepared to provide honest answers to questions concerning the patient's primary diagnosis, his or her level of alertness and physical mobility, skin problems, bladder control, and dietary requirements. Know whether the prospective resident will require physical, occupational, or speech therapy and whether he or she is oxygen dependent or on any artificial form of life support.

Many facilities accept patients for short-term or respite care. Is this what the family is considering, or are they seeking long-term care? Motivation for nursing home placement will also be explored. Does the prospective resident have any emotional disorders? Does he or she have a history of abusive behavior? Nursing homes are not permitted to admit persons who have proven to be a danger to themselves or to others. Abusive behavior on the part of the care recipient may prohibit admission to the facility.

Financial considerations will also be discussed. Many families are financially unprepared for nursing home placement. Many facilities accept private payment, Medicare, Medicaid, and Department of Veteran's Affairs (VA) benefits. A complete discussion of the Medicare and Medicaid programs appears in Chapter 12.

Florida nursing homes are licensed by the AHCA, which assigns either a "superior," "standard," or "conditional" rating to each licensed facility. Florida law requires that a facility's license be prominently displayed. The license will state the facility's rating status. A superior rating generally means that the facility offers quality nursing care in a clean and safe environment. It also means that the facility offers stimulating activities and other services that place it above other nursing homes in the community. The results of the facility's last state licensure survey should be available for your inspection. Keep in mind that appearances can be deceiving: a lavish facility may not necessarily signal good resident care.

One of the most important aspects of nursing home care is staffing. Most nursing homes employ a variety of staff to meet residents' needs. Inquire about the facility's medical director and what his or her responsibility is to residents. Many facilities require that residents be seen at least monthly by the medical director or by their own physicians. This may be preventative medicine in some cases, but may be medically necessary in others. The medical director is usually on call 24 hours a day and is a frequent visitor to the facility. He or she should have a good bedside manner and should be available to address residents' or family members' questions and concerns.

Most nursing homes employ registered nurses, licensed practical nurses, and nursing assistants on a 24-hour-a-day basis. Staffing ratios, the comparison of the number of nurses to the number of patients, are extremely important and should be addressed during the course of your visit, along with the facility's staff turnover rate. A high turnover rate may mean that health care workers are overworked and underpaid or may signal a more serious problem with quality of care. A stable staff, particularly at the department head level, is a strong indicator of a consistent standard of care. Knowing who their nursing assistant will be on a daily basis is often comforting to residents and their family members.

Therapies offered in the nursing home setting are a major consideration for some prospective residents. Many facilities offer physical, occupational, and speech therapy. Others also offer respiratory therapy. If a resident's physician orders therapy, the individual can immediately be evaluated by the appropriate therapist, who can then work closely with the resident and family members toward established goals, such as ambulation or regaining the ability to speak after a stroke. In some cases, therapy may enable the resident to function independently and return to his or her home. If your loved one will be receiving physical therapy, it is a good idea to meet the therapist. Visit the therapy room and note the types of equipment used.

Food—taste, quantity, and attention to individual dietary needs—is a major concern. Nursing home residents are often on physician-prescribed diets that must be closely monitored by a dietitian and the nursing staff. Supplemental feedings are sometimes required, as are weight loss or weight gain diets. Patients using internal tube feeding, such as a nasalgastric tube or a gastrostomy tube, must be closely supervised. Some nursing homes do not admit patients who require intravenous feedings. Recreational therapy or activities departments perform a vital function in nursing homes, providing stimulating activities, from adult education programs and exercise, cooking and arts and crafts classes, to wine and cheese parties. Many facilities offer pet therapy and adopt-a-grandparent programs. Activities should be innovative and scheduled on a regular basis. Most importantly, residents should be actively involved in choosing the activities they wish to participate in, and the choices should be many and varied. Even bedridden and dementia patients can be included in activities. No matter how advanced an individual's illness may be, stimulation through friendly conversation or touch therapy may be the key to his or her well-being.

Community involvement can be a great asset to nursing home residents. By staying involved, residents with less severe restrictions on their activities can maintain their independence by participating in the clubs and civic organizations they enjoyed before becoming ill. This can help them adjust to nursing home life. Many facilities have buses or mini-vans that are available to transport residents to special events. When you tour the nursing home, ask residents if they enjoy available activity programs.

If a prospective resident has been active in a church or synagogue, it is important to determine whether non- or interdenominational religious services are available. In any nursing home, each resident must be afforded the opportunity to practice his or her religion. Residents should be encouraged and, if necessary, assisted by the staff in maintaining their religious liberties.

Many facilities employ full-time social workers. They can greatly assist new residents in adjusting to their surroundings and provide much-needed counseling to family members during the initial transition period. A social worker plays a critical role in shaping the nursing home experience, assisting residents in obtaining adaptive devices, such as hearing aids, dentures, or wheelchairs; providing grief counseling; and assisting in the organization of "family councils." These organizations, made up of nursing home residents' family members, meet monthly or quarterly to discuss issues that affect participants' loved ones. Family members may use this time to air suggestions or complaints or simply to get to know other families. There is no question that council members share a common bond. Every nursing home should have a family council as a complement to a "residents' council." Residents, too, should be encouraged to take an active part in the decision-making process at the facility in which they reside.

Pharmaceutical services are usually provided by a consulting pharmacist, with services billed to the resident. In some facilities, residents can continue to use their own pharmacies, provided that they operate according to state guidelines for nursing home services. Florida law prohibits family members from supplying pharmaceuticals to residents.

Ancillary services, such as beautician or barber services, should be available to residents at reasonable rates. For many women, a visit to the beauty salon can do wonders for self-esteem. Many nursing homes give families the option of doing their family member's personal laundry themselves or of letting the nursing home do it for a nominal fee.

When touring a facility look for the following:

- Smiling faces. Notice the interaction between the nursing home staff and residents and their visiting family members.
- Cleanliness. There should be no heavy odors, whether pleasant or offensive. A good home will not use highly scented disinfectants to mask odors.
- Ongoing recreational activities or discussion groups.
- Well-lit and clutter-free hallways. *You should not see residents unattended in hallways, sitting slumped over in their chairs.*

A good time to take a tour is during mealtime. When entering the dining room, notice whether the food looks and smells appetizing. Residents who need assistance with eating should be well-attended to. Ask residents if they enjoy the food. Better yet, seek out an invitation to lunch or dinner. If you do not like the food, chances are that your friend or loved one will not either. Inquire as to whether family members are permitted and/or encouraged to join residents at mealtime. Residents should also be permitted to go out with their families for meals if they choose.

Ask to see residents' rooms. A facility may have private, semi-private, or small group accommodations. Inquire as to whether residents are permitted to bring personal articles from home, such as a favorite easy chair or family photos. In many facilities, residents can decorate their rooms as they choose. While touring residents' accommodations, again look for cleanliness and a clutter-free environment. All rooms should include:

- a privacy curtain or screen for each bed
- separate closet space for each resident
- a call light near each bed that signals the need for assistance
- conveniently located bathroom facilities that offer privacy and easy access for wheelchairs. Showers, bathtubs, and the commode area should have support bars.

The decision regarding selection of a private versus a semi-private room may be clear cut or a close call, depending on the personality and health status of the prospective resident. Private rooms, very simply, offer privacy. But one person's privacy can be another's isolation. Semi-private rooms provide an opportunity for socialization and the development of new friendships. A compatible roommate can ease the trauma associated with the adjustment to nursing home life. Expect to pay a few dollars more per day for a private room.

If, after careful consideration, you, your loved one, and other family members determine that a particular nursing home is best suited to your needs, the question of availability of beds comes into the picture. *Many facilities have long waiting lists at certain times of the year.* If the facility you have chosen has an immediate opening, there are several steps that must be completed prior to admission.

To avoid inappropriate placement that could endanger your loved one's well-being, it is essential that the facility receive a thorough medical history from the attending physician. After the medical report is obtained, the director of nursing, along with the admissions coordinator or administrator, will determine whether placement is appropriate. The admissions coordinator will then contact the prospective resident or family members and apprise them of admission status. Florida law requires a recent physical (usually within 90 days preceding admission), a tuberculosis screen, and a tetanus booster shot prior to admission.

Nursing Home Residents' Rights

Nursing home residents' rights are clearly defined in state and federal law. The Florida Long-Term Care Ombudsman Council has published the following "Bill of Rights":

- Nursing home residents have the right to maintain civil and religious liberties.
- They should have knowledge of available choices, and independent personal decision, which will not be infringed upon, and the right to encouragement and assistance from staff in the fullest possible exercise of these rights.
- Residents have the right to receive private and uncensored communication.
- Residents have the right to manage their own finances or delegate this to the facility, which must provide the resident with a quarterly statement.
- Residents have the right to be informed in writing and orally of refund policy and service charges that are not covered under Medicare and Medicaid.
- They have the right to be informed about their own medical condition, proposed treatment, and the right to refuse medication or treatment.
- Residents have the right to be provided adequate health care, social, mental health, recreational, and rehabilitative services.
- Nursing home residents have the right to privacy during treatment and while caring for personal needs.
- They have the right to be treated courteously, fairly, and with dignity.
- Nursing home residents have the right to be free from mental and physical abuse and from physical and chemical restraint.

- Nursing home residents have the right to be transferred or discharged only for medical reasons, the welfare of other residents, or nonpayment of bills.
- They must have freedom of choice in selecting a physician, pharmacy, and community activities.
- They may retain and use personal clothing and possessions.
- They may also have a copy and explanation of the facility rules and must be informed of the bed reservations policy for the facility.

Anyone who reports a complaint concerning suspected violations of residents' rights or conditions in a facility is immune from criminal or civil liability unless he or she has acted in bad faith.

When visiting nursing homes, ask for a copy of each facility's "Resident Rights."

There are additional protections for Florida nursing home residents. If a you or a loved one has a question or a problem concerning his or her care that remains unresolved after it is brought to the attention of the facility, contact the Florida Long-Term Care Ombudsman Council in Tallahassee at (904) 488-6190 or the district council office located nearest you. A complete listing of district offices is included in Chapter 16.

Ombudsman Council members are appointed by the governor. Each council has up to 30 members, including health professionals, social workers, attorneys, and nursing home residents or consumer advocates. The councils are charged with working with nursing homes and other long-term care facilities to increase their responsiveness to the people they serve. When nursing home residents are unable to speak for themselves, ombudsmen will act in their behalf to see that they receive necessary assistance.

There are many things to consider when making your decision regarding nursing home placement. There is no question that it will be one of the most difficult decisions you and your loved one will ever make. You may not want to make the decision alone. As painful as it may be, it is essential that you involve your loved one unless he or she is severely mentally incapacitated. Family members should be included in the decision making to avoid second guessing after placement.

You can not pass off a nursing home as anything other than what it is: a new home, temporary for some, permanent for most. There is nothing more condescending or cruel to your loved one than to try to sugar coat the issue. If you cannot bring yourself to use the "N-word," find a counselor who can help you work through your anxieties. Your local *Elder Helpline* should be able to refer you to a social worker or psychologist who specializes in issues affecting the elderly. You may want to involve other family members and invite them to visit the facility so that they may see first-hand what it has to offer. In the best of circumstances, you should bring your loved one in for a preadmission visit to ease his or her fears concerning nursing home placement and to involve him in the decision-making.

Most facilities will allow a 30-day "trial period," during which older persons and their loved ones can adjust to a new and, often times, emotionally-charged situation without the added pressure of having to view the decision as cast in stone.

Nursing Home Checklist

- Is the nursing home conveniently located for family and friends?
- Is the general atmosphere in the nursing home friendly and supportive?
- Do you feel at ease when visiting the facility?
- What is the general attitude of the staff? Do they appear cooperative and supportive, both with each other and with residents?
- Do residents appear comfortable?
- What do residents or their family members think of the facility?
- What will the total monthly charges run, including all ancillary services? Will the facility accept whatever government financial assistance your loved one may receive as payment in full? Is a deposit required prior to placement, and under what circumstances will it be refunded?
- Have you been given an opportunity to review the nursing home contract?

The American Association of Homes for the Aging (AAHA), an industry group, has published an excellent pamphlet on the nursing home decision. "Choosing a Nursing Home: A Guide to Quality Care" is available by contacting AAHA at 901 E St., NW, Suite 500, Washington, DC 20004 or at (202) 783-2242.

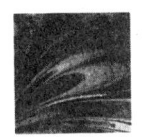

Profile

"Mac" and *"Noma"* worked all of their lives and are described by friends and family members as responsible, decent, God-fearing, tax-paying citizens.

Mac's Air Force career spanned 26 years, from World War II, through the Korean and Vietnam wars. He and Noma raised three children, putting all of them through college without government assistance. "We lived simply and saved money for our retirement," Noma says.

Mac and Noma bought health insurance, including long-term care insurance, and took comfort in the fact that Mac, who was diagnosed with Alzheimer's disease three years ago, would be eligible for care in a Veterans' Administration facility if the need arose.

But now they find that even though they took all possible precautions to avoid it, their savings will be wiped out by Mac's illness.

Because Mac has episodes of aggressive behavior and is an escape risk, he cannot be kept in a nursing home unless it has a locked unit. In attempting to find a space for Mac, Noma discovered that there is a waiting list for locked-unit beds. Mac currently is No. 6 on a list at a nearby facility, but the admissions director offers little hope that he will ever get to No. 1. Since there is no available bed, Mac's long-term care insurance will not pay for the cost of his care.

The only facility open to Mac is the geriatric long-term care facility at one of the state hospitals. There, he is housed with psychiatric patients and is the frequent victim of injuries since he is incapable of recognizing danger and how to avoid it. Each month, Noma writes a check for $2,000 to cover the cost of Mac's care. Because of

Mac's retirement income from the military, he will never become eligible for Medicaid.

"I see no bright cloud for either of us," Noma says. "He is the primary victim of this dreadful disease, but I am surely another."

Noma says that the pain has been agonizing as she has witnessed Mac's personhood disappear. She says that she has seen her once proud and strong Air Force chief master sergeant become a mumbling, shuffling body with no memory, no plans, no ideas, no control over his bodily functions, and no connection with his family or his environment.

Noma recently wrote a letter to President Clinton, appealing for assistance for herself and her family and for the countless other families caught in the hellish nightmare of a failed health care system.

"If the leaders of this country do not address this problem aggressively, now," she says, "thousands more families will experience the terrible despair that is our family's constant companion."

12

Medicare, Medicaid, and Medicare Supplement Insurance

Thomas Walter Poulton

It's a puzzle.

And, like all puzzles, arranging for the health care of a care recipient can be frustrating. Fortunately, there is a wide range of options for insurance and government assistance that can make the job easier.

Whether it is Medicaid, Medicare, or some type of private health insurance, remember to keep a few basic things in mind.

Make sure you have applied and been accepted *before* the care recipient needs medical treatment. Applying for a program at the time treatment is necessary can delay payment of medical bills. In many cases, it will be too late to have expenses associated with that treatment covered.

Make sure that you understand what is covered and what is not. The services covered by Medicare and Medicaid change every year. Keep in touch with government offices that can keep you updated on revisions.

Make sure that you keep all health care records, including correspondence from physicians and hospitals, statements of eligibility and coverage from Medicare, Medicaid, or your insurance company, and a record of any expenses you incur. These records may play a significant role in determining future eligibility and can be vital if you want to appeal a decision regarding coverage.

This chapter focuses on three sources of financial assistance, Medicare, Medicaid, and Medicare supplement, that are available to help meet the health care needs of your older loved one. The state and federal programs are confusing and sales pitches for Medicare supplement insurance policies can be misleading. But help is available.

The Florida Department of Elder Affairs (DOEA) in 1993 implemented the SHINE (Serving Health Insurance Needs of Elders) program in 16 counties that provides health insurance counseling to elders and their caregivers. Staffed by 200 elder volunteers, SHINE is specifically designed to provide answers to questions regarding Medicare, Medicaid and Medicare supplement insurance. Volunteers also help clients organize bills and paperwork and assist them in submitting claims and appeals.

SHINE counseling sessions are held at community facilities such as libraries, hospitals, and senior citizen centers. Appointments generally are required. To find out if there is a SHINE program in your area, contact your local *Elder Helpline*, A complete listing is included in Chapter 16.

There are many instances in which program eligibility overlaps. Medicaid, for example, may pay all or part of a person's Medicare insurance premium. Be sure to ask whether your care recipient can take advantage of these overlaps. But, in the case of supplemental insurance, make sure that you are not buying unnecessary coverage that duplicates what is already available through Medicare.

This chapter outlines many of the services available through Medicare and Medicaid during 1993. While some will remain unchanged in future years, you should always check with the appropriate agency to be sure of what is covered and what is not.

Following each program description in this chapter, you will find the current phone numbers for enrollment assistance and for program information. Those numbers are also subject to change. You may need to look through your local telephone directory for the correct number of the appropriate agency.

Medicare

Medicare is the most common source of payment for health care provided to the elderly in the United States. It is a federal government insurance program for which almost all persons aged 65 or older are eligible. Some persons, particularly the disabled, may be eligible before they turn 65.

Medicare is run by the Health Care Financing Administration of the U.S. Department of Health and Human Services. Applications and requests for information are handled by local Social Security Administration offices.

Medicare is composed of two parts, Part A and Part B.

PART A

Part A of the Medicare insurance program, known as Hospital Insurance, does not require a premium. It covers many of the costs associated with inpatient hospital care, some care in a skilled nursing facility, home health care, and hospice care.

A care recipient is eligible for Medicare Part A if he or she is aged 65 or older and

- receives benefits under the Social Security or Railroad Retirement systems, OR
- could receive benefits under the Social Security or Railroad Retirement systems but did not apply for them, OR
- if the recipient or the recipient's spouse had certain government employment.

If the care recipient is under 65 years of age, he or she may be eligible for Part A if he or she has been a Social Security or Railroad Retirement Board disability beneficiary for more than 24 months. Even if a disabled recipient cannot qualify for Medicare Part A through work history, it may be possible to pay a monthly premium and enroll in both Part A and Part B.

Certain government employees and their families may also be eligible for Medicare if they have been disabled for more than 29 months. Eligible persons should check with a local Social Security Administration office as soon as they become disabled.

Some persons are also eligible for Medicare Part A if they receive continuing dialysis for permanent kidney failure or if they have had a kidney transplant.

The amount that Medicare PART A will pay varies with what kind of care is needed and the amount of care already received.

Inpatient Hospital Care

Medicare Part A will pay for inpatient hospital services if all four of the following conditions are met: 1) a physician prescribes inpatient hospital care for an illness or injury; 2) the care required can be provided only by a hospital; 3) the hospital participates in Medicare (in some situations, Medicare will pay for emergency inpatient care in a nonparticipating hospital); and 4) a special review committee (a utilization review committee of the hospital or a peer review organization working for the Medicare program) does not disapprove the care recipient's stay.

If the four conditions are met, Medicare will pay for 90 days of medically necessary care in a given benefit period. A benefit period begins the first day a patient is admitted to the hospital and ends when the patient has not been in the hospital for a period of 60 consecutive days.

During 1993:

- Medicare paid all of the costs of inpatient care except for the first $676. The patient was responsible for paying this deductible. Hospitals could charge this deductible only for the first stay in a benefit period. In other words, if a patient was readmitted within the benefit period, the hospital could not charge a deductible for the second stay.
- For the 61st through the 90th day in each benefit period, Medicare pays for all covered services except for $169 a day. The patient is responsible for paying this hospital coinsurance.

You should be aware, however, that each Medicare participant is entitled to 60 inpatient reserve days in his or her lifetime. They can be used when a care recipient has exhausted the 90-day limit in a given benefit period. However, unlike the benefit period, they are not renewable. Once they have been used, no more reserve days are available to that care recipient.

During 1993:

- Medicare paid for all covered services except for $338 a day for each reserve day used.

Some of the major hospital inpatient services covered by Medicare are:

- a semiprivate room (a private room may be covered if it is medically necessary)
- all meals, including special diets
- regular nursing services (services of private nurses are not covered)

- special care units, such as intensive or coronary care units
- drugs furnished by the hospital during the recipient's stay;
- blood transfusions furnished by the hospital during the recipient's stay
- laboratory tests included in the hospital bill
- x-rays and other radiology services
- some medical supplies, such as casts and splints
- use of medical appliances, like a wheelchair
- operating and recovery room costs, including anesthesia; and
- rehabilitation services, such as physical and occupational therapy.

Medicare Part A will also pay for care in special hospitals and in a limited number of foreign hospitals.

For example, Medicare Part A will pay for 190 days of psychiatric hospital care in a person's lifetime. Once the 190 days have been used, however, Medicare will not pay for any more inpatient psychiatric hospital care.

It will also pay for care received in certain Mexican and Canadian hospitals under the following special circumstances: 1) the recipient is in the United States when an emergency occurs and a Canadian or Mexican hospital is closer than the nearest U.S. hospital that provides the needed services; or 2) the recipient lives in the United States and a Canadian or Mexican hospital is closer to the recipient than the nearest U.S. hospital that provides the services needed, regardless of whether there is an emergency situation

If the recipient is planning to travel outside the United States, check with a travel or insurance agent on the purchase of special short-term health insurance for foreign travel.

Nursing Homes

Medicare Part A will help pay for inpatient care at a Medicare-participating skilled nursing facility (SNF) following a hospital stay if the recipient's condition requires care that, for practical purposes, can be provided only in a skilled nursing facility.

Note, however, that many nursing homes are not licensed by the state as SNFs, and that many SNFs are not Medicare participants. To make matters more confusing, in some facilities, only a portion of the facility is designated as a Medicare facility. That is, some parts of a facility will accept Medicare while others will not. If a facility cannot tell you whether it participates or to what degree it participates, ask your Social Security office to check with the Health Care Financing Administration.

Medicare Part A helps pay for SNF care if five conditions are met: 1) the care recipient has been in a hospital at least three days in a row (not counting the day of discharge) before being transferred to the SNF; 2) admission to the SNF is required by a condition that was treated at the hospital; 3) admission occurs shortly after discharge from the hospital (usually within 30 days); 4) a physician certifies that the recipient needs and receives skilled nursing or rehabilitative care on a daily basis; and 5) a review committee does not disapprove your stay.

Part A will not pay for a stay in a skilled nursing facility unless the services provided there are needed on a daily basis. Also, it will not pay for such a facility if the recipient can cost effectively receive the needed care through some means other than a skilled nursing facility. Part A also does not pay for a recipient's stay if the main reason for being in a skilled nursing facility is to receive custodial care—services that can be delivered by lower-skilled health care workers.

If a recipient's stay in a skilled nursing facility is covered by Part A, Medicare will help pay for up to 100 days in a benefit period. During 1993, Medicare would pay all of the costs of covered services for the first 20 days. For the 21st through the 100th day, Medicare paid for all services except for $84.50 a day. The facility may charge the recipient up to that amount.

Physician services while in a nursing home may be covered by Medicare Part B. That portion of the Medicare program is described later in this chapter.

Some of the major SNF services covered by Medicare are:

- a semiprivate room
- all meals, including special diets
- regular nursing services (Medicare will not cover private duty nurses)
- rehabilitative services, such as physical, occupational, or speech therapy
- drugs furnished by the facility
- blood transfusions
- medical supplies, such as splints or casts
- use of appliances, such as a wheelchair.

Home Health Care

An alternative for many recipients who need skilled nursing care is a participating home health agency. Medicare Part A and Part B combine to pay much of the cost of skilled services provided by a home health agency if four conditions are met: 1) the care needed includes periodic skilled nursing care, physical therapy, or speech therapy; 2) the recipient is confined to the home; 3) a physician determines that the recipient needs home health care and sets up a home health plan; and 4) the home health agency providing care participates in the Medicare program.

Covered services do not include general household services, such as meal preparation or shopping. But they do include:

- part-time or intermittent skilled nursing care (usually up to eight hours of reasonable and necessary care per day for up to 21 consecutive days, longer in some circumstances)
- physical and speech therapy
- occupational therapy
- medical social services
- medical supplies
- most of the cost of durable medical equipment.

Hospice Care

A hospice is a facility that cares for terminally ill persons and their families. It specializes in treating pain and in offering supportive services to the terminally ill.

Medicare Part A will pay for hospice care if three conditions are met: 1) a physician certifies that a recipient is terminally ill; 2) the recipient chooses to receive care from a hospice rather than to receive the standard Medicare benefits; and 3) care is provided by a participating hospice.

Limitations on the benefit period for a hospice are different than for the benefit periods for hospital care or for a nursing home. Medicare Part A will pay for two 90-day periods and for one 30-day period, sometimes longer. Benefit periods may run consecutively. A recipient may also disenroll from a hospice and return to regular Medicare coverage, then re-elect hospice at another time (if there is a benefit period remaining). Even if the benefit periods expire, the hospice must continue to provide care. Under this circumstance, the hospice may bill the recipient for services rendered beyond the benefit periods.

Medicare pays for all of a hospice stay except for very small coinsurance amounts related to outpatient drugs and inpatient respite care.

During 1993, the recipient paid 5 percent of the cost of outpatient drugs or $5 for each prescription, whichever was less. The recipient also paid 5 percent of the Medicare rate for inpatient respite care (approximately $4.48 a day).

Medicare Part A does not pay for hospice treatments unrelated to pain relief or symptom management.
Covered hospice services are:

- nursing services
- physician services
- drugs, including outpatient prescriptions
- physical, occupational and speech therapy
- home health aide and homemaker services
- medical social services
- medical supplies and appliances
- short-term inpatient care, respite care
- counseling.

Questions about services or claims covered under Medicare Part A should be directed to the Medicare intermediaries. In Florida, the intermediaries are Blue Cross and Blue Shield, P.O. Box 2711, Jacksonville, FL 32231, (904) 363-0632; Mutual of Omaha, P.O. Box 1602, Omaha, NE, 68101, (402) 978-2860; and Aetna, 25400 U.S. Hwy. 19 North, Suite 135, Clearwater, FL, 34623, (813) 796-8292.

PART B

Medicare Part B, known as Supplementary Medical Insurance, is the portion of the Medicare program that helps pay for physician and outpatient services. It also helps pay for dentist, optometrist, and certain home health services.

Most of the people enrolled in Medicare Part B pay a monthly premium ($36.60 in 1993) and a yearly deductible of $100. In addition, every time a recipient uses a service he or she may be required to pay a coinsurance amount.

Low-income individuals may be able to have their state's Medicaid program pay for the Part B premium. Some may even be designated as qualified Medicare beneficiaries. Such recipients may be able to get their Medicaid programs to pay all of their costs not picked up by Medicare, including coinsurance and deductibles.

Any person who is eligible for the premium-free Part A component of Medicare, based on the work-related conditions noted earlier in this chapter, may enroll in Part B. Even if a recipient cannot qualify for Medicare Part A, it may be possible to pay a monthly premium and enroll in both Part A and Part B.

Deductibles and Coinsurance

During 1993, a recipient was responsible for paying the first $100 of Medicare-covered services. The deductible must be met only once every year and can be met through paying for any combination of services.

After the deductible amount has been paid, a recipient must also pay a coinsurance amount (a percentage of the Medicare charge for covered services, usually 20 percent).

Some providers will accept the amount Medicare pays as payment in full. This is called providing services "on assignment." But if a provider charges more than Medicare approves for a service, the recipient must pay the 20 percent coinsurance, plus any amount over the approved amount.

For example, let us suppose that Dr. Smith performs a service for Mrs. Jones and charges $1,500. If Mrs. Jones has paid her $100 deductible for the year, and if Medicare's approved rate for the service was $1,100, Mrs. Jones would have to pay $220, representing the 20 percent of the $1,100 Medicare-approved amount, plus the $400 difference between what Dr. Smith charges and the approved amount.

Mrs. Jones would pay a total of $620 for the services provided by Dr. Smith. Medicare would pay $880, representing 80 percent of the $1,100 approved by Medicare.

Finding a physician who takes assignment can save time as well as money. Physicians who take assignment will usually handle all of the claims paperwork, charging the recipient for any part of the $100 deductible not yet met, the 20 percent coinsurance amount, and for any services not covered by Medicare.

Two new Medicare rules should be noted. First, all physicians and medical suppliers must fill out claims forms for patients and mail them to Medicare, regardless of whether they take assignment. Second, physicians are prohibited from charging more than the assignment rate for services rendered to persons who qualify for their state's Medicaid program.

If possible, before receiving services, the recipient or the caregiver should ask a provider if he or she will accept Medicare assignment.

Physician Services

There are many types of physicians whose services are covered by Medicare Part B, including doctors of medicine, osteopathy, podiatric medicine, dental surgery or dental medicine, and optometry. The services of chiropractors are also covered by Medicare Part B.

The major services covered are:

- medical and surgical, including anesthesia
- diagnostic tests and procedures that are part of treatment
- radiology and pathology services while the recipient is a hospital inpatient or outpatient
- treatment of mental illness (more limited if provided on an outpatient basis)
- services performed in a physician's office, such as x-rays; nurses; blood transfusions; medical supplies; and physical, occupational and speech pathology services.

Services not covered include:

- routine physical examinations and tests related to such examinations (some PAP smears are covered, however)
- most routine foot care
- examinations for prescribing or fitting eyeglasses or hearing aids
- immunizations, except for some pneumococcal vaccinations or immunizations and Hepatitis B for certain at-risk persons
- most cosmetic surgery.

Chiropractic Services

Medicare helps pay for only one kind of treatment by a licensed chiropractor—the manual manipulation of the spine to correct an irregularity that can be demonstrated by an x-ray. Medicare Part B does not pay for other diagnostic or therapeutic services, including x-rays, furnished by a chiropractor.

Podiatric services

Medicare Part B helps pay for the covered services of a podiatrist. These commonly include treatment for ingrown toenails, hammer toe or bunion deformities, and heel spurs. Medicare Part B generally does not cover routine foot care such as the cutting or removal of corns or calluses, trimming of nails, or other hygienic care.

It will cover some routine services, however, for recipients suffering from a medical condition that requires a podiatrist, an osteopath, or a doctor of medicine to treat the routine condition.

Dental Services

Medicare does not cover care related to the treatment, filling, removal, or replacement of teeth. Nor does it cover root canal therapy or surgery or surgery for impacted teeth. Medicare does help pay for the services of a dentist in certain cases where a medical problem is related to a dental condition. If dental work requires hospitalization, Medicare Part A will pay for the recipient's hospital stay even if the dental care is not covered by Part B. Medicare does not pay for dental plates or other dental devices.

Optometric Services

Medicare helps pay for some of the services performed by optometrists but only if the optometrist is legally authorized by the state to provide those services. Medicare will not pay for routine eye exams or for eyeglasses and corrective lenses (it may pay for corrective lenses, however, if they are prosthetic and replace the natural lens of the eye).

Medicare Part B also covers the services of a variety of special practitioners, including certified registered nurse anesthetists, certified nurse midwives, physician assistants, and clinical psychologists.

For surgical procedures, many recipients may want to consider getting a second opinion. Medicare will pay for a second opinion in many circumstances. Contact your Medicare intermediary for more information on second opinions.

Outpatient Hospital Services

Medicare Part B will help pay for covered services a person receives as an outpatient at a Medicare-participating hospital. It will also pay for some emergency services at nonparticipating hospitals.

When a recipient is treated in an outpatient setting, the health care provider is likely to ask how much of the $100 Medicare Part B deductible has been met. One easy way to demonstrate a recipient's having paid all or a portion of that deductible is to show the provider the recipient's most recent *Explanation of Medicare Benefits* notice, which is mailed to the recipient every time Medicare is used.

If the hospital cannot tell how much of the deductible has been paid and the bill is less than $100, it might ask the recipient to pay the entire bill. If a recipient pays the bill but has already met the deductible, the insurance company acting as Medicare's carrier or the hospital will refund the amount overpaid.

Medicare Part B will help pay for the following major outpatient services:

- services provided in an emergency room or outpatient clinic, including ambulatory surgical procedures
- lab tests included in the hospital bill
- mental health care in an outpatient hospital psychiatric program when a physician certifies that inpatient services would be required without it
- x-rays and other radiology services billed by the hospital
- medical supplies such as splints and casts
- certain drugs and biologicals
- blood transfusions.

Medicare Part B also will help pay for a limited range and cost of other health care services, including ambulatory surgical services.

Medicare Part B will help pay for some surgical procedures at an ambulatory surgical center, including the costs associated with physicians' and anesthesia services. To be covered, however, such procedures and services must be performed at ambulatory surgical centers that have entered into agreements with Medicare to provide the services.

Home Health Services

If a recipient has Part B of Medicare but does not have Part A, Medicare Part B will pay for the same home health care services previously described.

Outpatient Physical and Occupational Therapy and Speech Pathology Services

Medicare Part B will help pay for these services if three conditions are met: 1) the recipient's physician prescribes the services; 2) the recipient's physician or therapist sets up the plan of treatment to be used for these services; and 3) the recipient's physician periodically reviews the treatment plan.

These services may be received as an outpatient of a participating hospital or skilled nursing facility or from a participating home health agency, rehabilitation agency, or public health agency. In such cases, the provider will submit the claim form and may charge the recipient only for the unmet portion of the $100 deductible, the 20 percent share of the Medicare-approved amount, and noncovered services.

Another option is to receive these services from an independently practicing physical or occupational therapist. During 1993, Medicare Part B paid a maximum of $600 a year for services from such independent practitioners and only if the providers have been approved by the Medicare program.

AMBULANCE TRANSPORTATION

Medicare Part B will help pay for ambulance services if the ambulance, equipment, and personnel meet Medicare requirements and if transportation in another vehicle would endanger the recipient's health.

Ambulance services are paid for only if used for transportation to a hospital or skilled nursing facility or from a hospital or skilled nursing facility to the recipient's home. Medicare will also help pay for ambulance transportation from one facility to another if it is medically necessary to do so.

Medicare will not pay for ambulance service from the recipient's home to a doctor's office.

Durable Medical Equipment

Medicare Part B will help pay for durable medical equipment prescribed by a physician for use in the home, including oxygen and wheelchairs.

Most of the medical equipment Medicare pays for must be used on a rental basis, but Medicare will help pay for the purchase of some pieces of equipment.

Medicare Part B will also help pay for other types of services, such as: kidney dialysis and transplants, rural health clinic services, portable diagnostic x-ray services, radiation therapy, prosthetic devices, and comprehensive outpatient rehabilitation facility services.

After the recipient or a provider sends in a Part B claim, Medicare will mail to the recipient an *Explanation of Medicare Benefits* notice, which describes Medicare's decision on the claim. For the services of a physician, the notice will list covered services along with the Medicare-approved charge for those services, how much was paid by Medicare, and the status of the recipient's $100 deductible.

If there is a question about the benefits notice, call or write the Florida Medicare carrier. In 1993, the carrier was Medicare/Blue Shield of Florida, P.O. Box 2360, Jacksonville, FL 32231.

If you have brief questions about Medicare, such as the status of claims, or for copies of benefits notices, call (800) 666-7586. For other Medicare needs call (800) 333-7586 or (904) 355-3680.

RIGHT OF APPEAL

Appeal under Part A

There are many levels of appeal for the Medicare program and it is important that the correct procedure be followed if you or the care recipient wish to appeal a decision.

For Medicare Part A claims (such as hospital or ambulatory surgical center services), the first notice of noncoverage may come from the provider. This is not an official Medicare determination but you can ask the provider to get one. If you or the care recipient asks for an official determination, the provider must file a claim for the recipient. When the official determination arrives, and if the recipient still disagrees with the decision, the recipient may appeal.

When admitted for care to a hospital or ambulatory surgical center, the patient should receive a copy of *An Important Message From Medicare*. This publication will list and explain the duties of peer review organizations (PROs).

A peer review organization is a firm hired by the federal government to review the treatment provided to Medicare participants at hospitals and ambulatory surgical canters. PROs review Medicare claims as well as complaints from patients about the quality of care they receive.

If the recipient disagrees with the decision of a PRO, he or she may ask for a reconsideration. If the reconsideration decision is not satisfactory and the amount in question is $200 or more, the recipient can request a hearing from an administrative law judge. A case involving $2,000 or more can eventually make its way to a federal appellate court.

If elective or nonemergency surgery is at issue, the hospital or the PRO may become involved prior to admission. If the hospital believes that the claim will not be paid by Medicare, it may refuse admission without consulting the PRO. To do this, the hospital must put its decision in writing. If you or the care recipient disagree with such a decision, make a request to the PRO for immediate review. The request must be made to the PRO within three calendar days after receipt of the notice from the hospital.

In 1993, Florida's PRO was Blue Cross and Blue Shield of Florida, PRO Review, P.O. Box 45267, Jacksonville, FL, 32232-5785, (904) 791-8262.

Appeals of most of the other decisions in Medicare Part A (such as skilled nursing facilities, home health care, or hospice services) are handled by the Medicare intermediary. The Medicare intermediary is an insurance company hired by the federal government to administer Part A of Medicare. If you or a care recipient wishes to appeal the decision of an intermediary, you have 60 days from the date you receive the initial decision to request reconsideration. The request can be sent directly to the intermediary or through the Social Security Administration.

If you or the recipient disagree with the reconsideration decision and the amount in dispute is at least $100, you may request a hearing from an administrative law judge. If the case involves $1,000 or more it may eventually be heard in federal appellate court.

Appeal under Part B

Every time a care recipient or a Part B provider files a Medicare claim, the recipient will be sent An Explanation of Medicare Benefits notice. The notice will describe the charges covered by Medicare and explain the process for appealing a decision.

If the recipient disagrees with the decision on the claim, he or she may, within six months of receiving the decision, ask for a review by the carrier. If the review decision is still not satisfactory and involves at least $100, the recipient may ask for a hearing before the hearing officer for the carrier. The decision of the hearing officer may be appealed to an administrative law judge if it involves $500 or more.

Additional information about appeals is available from three sources: the Social Security Administration, Florida's Medicare carrier, or from a peer review organization.

ENROLLMENT IN MEDICARE

Enrolling in the Medicare program should generally be done as soon as the care recipient is eligible. This is a complicated process in some instances, particularly if the recipient is covered by health insurance. Failure to enroll at the first opportunity can delay eligibility for coverage and increase premiums. Questions should be immediately directed to the Social Security Administration.

Automatic Enrollment

If the recipient is getting Social Security or Railroad Retirement payments when he or she turns 65, he or she will automatically receive a Medicare card in the mail. The card will explain that the recipient can get both Medicare Part A and Part B. If the recipient does not want to participate in Part B, he or she should follow the instructions that come with the card.

The card will show which coverages (Part A and/or Part B) the recipient has and the date the coverage started. Always keep this card with the care recipient, particularly when traveling. It is also important to show this card any time the care recipient is receiving health care. If it is lost, contact Social Security immediately to get a new one. Never let anyone else use the Medicare card.

APPLYING FOR MEDICARE

If the care recipient does not automatically qualify for coverage, it may be possible to apply for, and enroll in, Part A and Part B. An application must be filled out for either part of Medicare if the recipient is:

- not receiving Social Security or Railroad Retirement benefits, OR
- if government employment is involved, OR
- if the recipient has kidney disease.

If enrollment will be based upon eligibility for Social Security, call the Social Security Administration. If enrollment is to be based upon eligibility for Railroad Retirement benefits, Florida residents should call the Railroad Retirement Board at (800) 833-4455.

If the recipient must apply for Medicare Part B, he should do so in what is called the seven-month "initial enrollment period." The starting date of the initial enrollment period will vary, depending on the basis of your eligibility. The recipient should apply within the first three months of the initial enrollment period to avoid delays in coverage.

Failure to enroll at any time during the initial enrollment period could delay coverage for up to 14 months and will probably result in a surcharge on the Medicare Part B premium.

With some exceptions, those who delay in enrolling will have to apply during a general enrollment period held from January 1 to March 31 each year. Coverage for people enrolling during this period will begin on the following July 1. Part B premiums will generally be 10 percent higher for each year the recipient could have been enrolled but was not.

If the recipient does not meet the Part A requirements for automatic eligibility but has Part B insurance, he or she can apply for Part A benefits and pay a special premium (in 1993, the premium for Part A was $221 a month). To buy Part A insurance, the recipient will probably be required to buy Part B insurance.

Those applying for Medicare Part A also have a general enrollment period from January 1 to March 31 each year. Again, failure to enroll during the first period for which the recipient is eligible may mean delays in coverage and increases in the premium.

Special Enrollment for those Already Insured

If the recipient is covered by an employer health plan related to current employment, he or she may be able to delay enrollment in Part A or Part B without paying a premium penalty and without waiting for a general enrollment period. Contact the Social Security Administration if this may apply to your care recipient.

CHANGES IN ELIGIBILITY

If the recipient has Medicare Part A as a result of the husband's or wife's employment history, that coverage will end if the recipient is divorced before the marriage has lasted 10 years.

A recipient who is buying Medicare Part A will lose that option if the recipient decides to cancel Part B. A recipient who buys Part A insurance must also enroll and pay the premium for Part B.

Disabled persons under age 65 who recover from their disabilities will lose their coverage. A disabled recipient who goes back to work will not lose Part A or Part B coverage for at least 48 months after returning to work if the applicable premiums are paid, however.

CLAIMS FOR A RECIPIENT WHO DIES

Any Part A payments due when a recipient dies are paid directly to the facility owed. Part B claims, however, may be paid to the estate if the recipient or the recipient's estate paid the bill.

PREPAID HEALTH CARE PLANS

Some health maintenance organizations (HMOs) and competitive medical plans (CMPs) are under contract with Medicare to provide services to participants. Most of these provide all of the services covered by Medicare and can do so in a time- and cost-efficient way. Some even provide additional services over and above what Medicare covers at little or no cost.

For information about an HMO's or CMP's participation in Medicare, contact the organization directly. They usually advertise when enrollment in their plan is open to Medicare beneficiaries.

The majority of the information in the Medicare section of this chapter comes from the 1993 edition of *The Medicare Handbook*. A copy of the latest edition of this very helpful book can be obtained from the Social Security Administration.

For additional information on Medicare, call (800) 333-7586.

Medicaid

Medicaid is a joint federal and state program that assists low-income persons in paying for the health care they need. Generally, it is designed to help the poorest people get the minimum levels of care they could not otherwise afford. But even some moderate-income people can qualify for help in paying very large bills. Do not count your care recipient out of this program until you have received a declaration of eligibility from the state Medicaid office. In 1985, almost 22 million people in the United States had at least a portion of their medical bills paid by Medicaid.

Like Medicare, Florida's Medicaid program is a maze of eligibility requirements and coverage limitations. The program is constantly changing and you should monitor these changes in the event your care recipient is affected.

A few of the key differences between Medicare and Medicaid are:

- Medicaid pays the provider directly
- the provider must accept Medicaid as payment in full
- Medicaid does not reimburse the recipient for payments made to providers.

A few of the key similarities are:

- not all providers accept Medicaid. In fact, far fewer accept Medicaid than accept Medicare

- both are government-run programs
- some of the services covered by Medicaid depend on age as well as income and assets.

APPLYING FOR MEDICAID

There are more than 500 Medicaid determination offices statewide, and which office you will deal with depends of the type of assistance you may be seeking (i.e., Medicaid nursing home or community care) and your or your loved one's precise street address. To complicate matters further, some, but not all, of the functions of the Medicaid program were transferred to the Agency for Health Care Administration, effective July 1, 1993.

In the short-term, the Department of Health and Rehabilitative Services (HRS) Aging and Adult Services district offices were expected to retain the oversight function for the Medicaid determination program. Legislative proposals were expected, however, that would transfer many of the remaining Aging and Adult Services programs to the Department of Elder Affairs. We've included a listing of the Aging and Adult Services district human services program offices in Chapter 16, but, again, your best bet avoiding wrong turns and dead ends is your local for *Elder Helpline*.

To apply for Medicaid, you or the recipient should call the office that you are referred to by the *Elder Helpline*. A worker there will help you arrange to fill out the necessary paperwork and to set an appointment for an interview. The recipient may need to bring several documents, including the following:

- a birth certificate
- pay stubs
- bank books
- medical bills
- Social Security card
- insurance policies.

It also is important to note that eligibility asset and income requirements for couples differ than those for single persons. It may, therefore, be necessary to bring some of these documents for a spouse, too.

Federal law requires that Medicaid determinations be completed within 45 days of the date of application. But case load backlogs, computer snafus and the complexity of the documentation required have resulted in waits of up to nine months in some parts of the state. If the applicant is deemed eligible for Medicaid assistance, some benefits will be paid retroactively to the date of application. If an application is denied because of income level, the denial notice will tell the recipient how high his or her medical bills must be for Medicaid to pay a share of them.

If you or the care recipient disagrees with the eligibility determination, you may ask for a hearing. To request a hearing, call or write the office that processed your application. At the hearing, anyone can represent the recipient, including the caregiver or an attorney.

To maintain your care recipient's eligibility, make sure you notify HRS of any changes in the recipient's address, medical condition, income or earnings, assets, employment, or living arrangements.

Assets that will be used to calculate eligibility determination include bank accounts, stocks and bonds, life insurance, and some property. However, the home in which the recipient lives is excluded from the assets determination. In 1993, up to $2,500 set aside for burial could also be excluded in the calculation of an individual's assets.

The following services, within certain limits, are covered by the Medicaid program:

- inpatient hospital services
- outpatient hospital services
- physician services
- laboratory and x-ray services
- skilled and intermediate care nursing home services
- home health care
- rural health clinic care
- medically necessary transportation
- prescribed drugs
- tate mental health hospital care
- intermediate care for the mentally retarded
- advanced registered nurse practitioner care
- dentures
- orthodontic services
- vision and hearing services, in some circumstances
- community mental health services
- podiatric services
- ambulatory surgical center care
- birthing center care

- hospice services
- Medicare premiums, deductibles, and coinsurance.

These services may be limited by the method used to qualify for Medicaid coverage. Payment for nursing home care, for example, is not available to individuals who qualify under the Medically Needy Program.

Also, the rules for the payment of Medicare premiums, deductibles, and coinsurance change frequently at both the federal and state levels. It is very important to keep up with these changes so that your care recipient does not miss paying a premium he or she did not previously have to pay.

SSI-RELATED PROGRAMS

There are eight public assistance programs for the aged, blind or disabled—called SSI-related programs in addition to the base Medicaid program: 1) Supplemental Security Income (SSI); 2) Medicaid Expansion Designated by SOBRA (MEDS-AD); 3) Qualified Medicare Beneficiaries (QMB); 4) Special Low-Income Medicare Beneficiary (SLMB); 5) the Medically Needy Program; 6) the Institutional Care Program (ICP); 7) Medicaid Hospice; and 8) the Optional State Supplementation Program (OSS).

Supplemental Security Income (SSI)

The SSI program was created to provide cash assistance to needy individuals in the community (as opposed to those in an institutional setting). If your care recipient qualifies for SSI payments, then he or she automatically qualifies for the Medicaid program. SSI recipients who need nursing home care must meet additional eligibility criteria to qualify for institutional benefits.

The following are the requirements for the SSI program (with the applicable 1993 dollar amounts listed in parentheses). An individual must:

- be at least 65 years of age, blind, or disabled;
- be a citizen or alien admitted for permanent residence;
- have assets below a certain amount ($2,000 in 1993);

- have monthly income below a certain amount (in 1993, $434 for individuals in their own households or $30 for individuals in nursing homes. Social Security payments are considered income); AND
- apply for all other benefits for which he or she may be eligible.

Payment is based upon how much income the individual or couple has and the amount of the current maximum payment standard. To apply for cash SSI payments, you or the care recipient should contact your local Social Security office.

Medicaid Expansion Designated by SOBRA (MEDS-AD)

MEDS-AD is designed to allow aged or disabled persons with incomes less than 90 percent of the federal poverty level to receive Medicaid coverage.

Your aged or disabled care recipient may be eligible for MEDS-AD if he or she:

- is at least 65 years of age or disabled;
- is a citizen or alien admitted for permanent residence;
- has assets below a certain level ($5,000 in 1993);
- has monthly income below a certain level ($523 in 1993); AND
- is applying for all other benefits for which he or she may be eligible.

To apply for MEDS-AD benefits, contact the *Elder Helpline* for referral to the appropriate local Aging and Adult Services office.

Qualified Medicare Beneficiaries (QMB)

This program entitles certain individuals who are either enrolled or conditionally enrolled in Medicare Part A to receive Medicare cost-sharing benefits, including payment of Medicare premiums, deductibles, and coinsurance. To be eligible, an individual must:

- be a citizen or alien admitted for permanent residence;
- have assets below a certain level ($5,000 in 1993);
- have monthly income below a certain level ($581 in 1993); AND
- be applying for all other benefits for which he or she may be eligible.

These benefits are paid only to providers who will accept Medicaid and are paid directly to them. Individuals cannot be reimbursed by Medicaid. To apply for QMB benefits, contact the *Elder Helpline* for referral to the appropriate local Aging and Adult Services office.

Special Low-Income Medicare Beneficiary (SLMB)

Through the SLMB program, Medicaid pays Medicare directly for eligible individuals' Medicare Part B premium. This "buy-in" benefit takes effect about three months after the individual receives notice of his or her SLMB application approval. To be eligible for SLMB benefits, individuals must:

- be enrolled or conditionally enrolled in Medicare Part A;
- be a citizen or alien admitted for permanent residence;
- have assets below a certain level ($5,000 in 1993);
- have gross monthly income below a certain level ($639 in 1993); AND
- be applying for all other benefits for which he or she may be eligible.

To apply for SLMB benefits, contact the *Elder Helpline* for referral to the appropriate local Aging and Adult Services office.

The Medically Needy Program

The purpose of the Medically Needy Program is to provide assistance with medical costs when an individual's medical expenses comes close to or exceed his or her income. There is no monthly income limit for eligibility as long as the individual has sufficient medical bills to bring his or her income down to a certain limit ($180 in 1993). Once the individual's medical bills reach the point where they are equal to or more than the individual's share of cost, the individual becomes eligible for Medicaid for that month. Medicaid will not pay for the bills that are used to meet the share of cost.

To be eligible, the individual must:

- be aged, disabled, or blind;
- be a citizen or alien admitted for permanent residence;
- have assets below a certain level ($5,000 in 1993);
- apply for all other benefits for which he or she may be eligible; AND

- meet the monthly share of cost.

To apply for benefits through the Medically Needy Program, contact the *Elder Helpline* for referral to the appropriate local Aging and Adult Services office.

The Institutional Care Program (ICP)

ICP is a medical assistance program that helps persons in nursing homes pay for the cost of nursing home care. To be eligible, an individual must:

- be at least 65 years of age, blind, or disabled;
- be a citizen or alien admitted for permanent residence;
- have assets below a certain level ($2,000 in 1993);
- have monthly income below a certain level ($1,302 in 1991);
- apply for all other benefits for which he or she may be eligible;
- be in medical need of nursing home care as determined by Aging and Adult Services or the appropriate state agency; AND
- be placed in a licensed Medicaid nursing home.

ICP operates differently from other programs in the way that it pays for services. Under ICP, almost all of the recipient's monthly income must be paid to the nursing home. The recipient is allowed to keep $35 a month for a personal needs allowance and, in some circumstances, an additional amount for the support of a spouse and dependents. Medicaid then pays the difference between what the recipient has paid the nursing home and the total amount the state has set for reimbursement to that nursing home. Veterans may be able to keep up to $90 a month of their income.

Medicaid Hospice

The Hospice program is a medical assistance program that maintains terminally ill individuals in their homes for as long as possible, avoiding institutionalization whenever possible.

Like the ICP program, all but a set amount of a patient's monthly income ($581 in 1993) must be applied to the hospice monthly charge for his or her care. Medicaid then pays the difference between the amount the patient is responsible for and the amount charged by the hospice.

To be eligible, the aged or disabled individual must:

- have a medical prognosis of terminally ill with a life expectancy of six months or less (certification of this prognosis by the medical provider satisfies the disability requirement);
- be a citizen or alien admitted for permanent residence;
- have assets below a certain level ($2,000 in 1993);
- have monthly income below a certain level ($1,302 in 1993);
- sign a hospice election statement, which says that he or she has selected hospice to the exclusion of regular Medicaid services; AND
- apply for all other benefits for which he or she may be eligible.

Participating hospice providers initiate the application process by obtaining the medical prognosis from the doctor and the election statement from the individual. Contact your local *Elder Helpline* for additional information.

Optional State Supplementation Program (OSS)

OSS is a cash assistance program designed to supplement an individual's income so that the individual can reside in a community alternative living arrangement and avoid institutionalization in a nursing home.

To be eligible, a recipient must:

- be at least 18 years of age;
- be aged, disabled, or blind;
- be a citizen or alien admitted for permanent residence;
- have assets below a certain level ($2,000 in 1993);
- have monthly income below a certain level ($575 in 1993);
- apply for all other benefits for which he or she may be eligible; AND
- be certified by Aging and Adult Services as needing placement in one of the following Agency for Health Care Administration (AHCA)-licensed facilities: adult foster care, adult congregate living facility (ACLF), home for special services, or mental health residential treatment facility.

Payment to the provider is on a basis similar to that described previously for ICP. Recipients are allowed a $43 monthly needs allowance.

Medicare Supplement Insurance

Medicare supplement insurance, also known as "medigap" insurance, may be a desirable option for your care recipient. If chosen wisely, a Medicare supplement policy can fill in the holes of Medicare coverage, both in terms of increasing the range of services covered and in helping to pay for those services. But many of these policies are unnecessary and duplicative of Medicare coverage. Some are even designed so that they offer very little or no protection beyond what Medicare has to offer. Others are simply worthless, their promoters hoping to take advantage of the confusion an older person faces in keeping up with the Medicare program.

Florida's Department of Insurance (DOI) has established a consumer hotline ((800) 342-2762) that can help answer some of the questions you or your care recipient may have when considering a supplemental policy. DOI personnel at this number can tell you whether an insurer is licensed in the state to sell Medicare supplement insurance. This can be important, because the department monitors these companies and their advertising to reduce deceptive practices.

Everyone's situation is unique and there is a wide range of insurance policies in the marketplace, but here are a few basic rules to follow when shopping for a Medicare supplement policy.

If your care recipient qualifies for both Medicare and Medicaid, he or she almost certainly does not need Medicare supplement insurance.

It may be to your care recipient's benefit to continue a group health insurance policy after retirement. This has the benefit of avoiding a period of noncoverage for any pre-existing conditions. Check with the employer to determine whether continuation is an option.

Rates and coverage vary a great deal. Compare the policies and prices carefully. If everything is not set out in writing, don't buy the policy.

Make sure that there is an easy-to-reach contact person in the event you have questions about a policy. Mail order policies, in particular, may lack local agents or toll-free telephone numbers.

Be aware of maximum benefits. Most policies have limits on the total amount they will pay or on the number of days for which they will pay.

Do not be pressured into purchasing a policy.

Complete the application for insurance carefully and accurately. Failure to do so may result in the company refusing to pay a claim or canceling coverage.

Make sure that you obtain and carefully read a clearly worded written summary of the policy.

Be wary of deceptive advertising techniques: a red, white, and blue envelope may look official, but the government has not and will not sponsor or endorse Medicare supplement insurance companies. Do not believe agents or advertisements that imply government sponsorship.

Use your 30-day free look option. You have 30 days to review a policy. If you or the recipient decides that the policy is inappropriate, send it back by certified or registered mail with the return receipt requested. This will make it easier to obtain a refund if you choose not to keep the policy.

For more information on how to shop for a Medicare supplement insurance policy, call the DOI consumer service office nearest you. A complete listing of these consumer service offices is included in Chapter 16.

The Corporate Response to Caregiving

Marie E. Cowart, R.N., Ph.D.

Annette, a receptionist for a medium-sized law firm, was 45 minutes late for work last Tuesday. She is spending an inordinate amount of time on the telephone dealing with personal business during working hours. About six months ago, she began calling in sick every other week. Of course, she has plenty of sick time after 20 years of employment during which she seldom was absent. But last Friday she let the telephone go unanswered while she completed a personal call on the other line. She is beginning to make mistakes and, when counseled, becomes angry and attacking. Her usual jovial nature has disappeared. Yet last year she received the annual outstanding employee award.

Annette is not job hunting. She is not an alcoholic. She is the primary caregiver of an older family member who lives in her household.

More and more employers are encountering this relatively new employee problem: the responsibility of caring for an older family member.

Dr. Robyn Stone of the National Center for Health Services Research conducted the first national survey of caregivers of the frail elderly in 1982. She learned that:

- One-third of caregivers are working, and almost three-quarters of caregivers are women—daughters and wives.
- Sometimes the caregiver is the husband. This is more likely to be the case in a couple's later years.

- Most caregivers are in their fifties. Some still have dependent children in the home in addition to the care recipient.
- Many caregivers, especially those at the lower income levels, serve as the sole provider of care with no outside assistance.
- Most care recipients are women in their late seventies. Many are over 85 years of age. In our later years, we are becoming a nation of women caring for women.

More than 13 million Americans—one in every six persons aged 45-64—are caring for an elderly parent or spouse. A third of all caregivers are employed and more than seven million workers have a disabled parent or spouse. Most working caregivers are women in low-paying hourly positions that afford little flexibility. Women in higher-status jobs are better able to establish flexible work schedules, to bring work home, or to purchase support services.

Restrictive Medicaid eligibility contributes to the fact that the low-middle class family, which is not eligible for Medicaid nursing home care and does not have the resources to pay for outside assistance, assumes the burden of personal care for a family member more often than other income groups. This situation has tremendous implications for businesses, especially those that have large numbers of low-wage women workers. Compounding the problem is the projected shrinking of the younger work force and an increasingly older population with a greater demand for caregiving.

Employer Initiatives

THE TRAVELLERS SURVEY

The Hartford-based Travelers Insurance Companies in 1985 surveyed its over-30 work force in 1985 to learn more about their employees' caregiving responsibilities. About 28 percent of employee respondents indicated they had caregiving responsibilities. Most were providing care to their mothers, although fathers and in-laws also received care. Many lived in the same house as their dependent family member and had younger children living in the home. This was even more likely when the caregiver was under age 55. A major illness, hospitalization, or the death of a spouse-caregiver most often precipitated the need for care.

Caregiving consisted of providing companionship and transportation, performing household chores like cleaning and cooking, coordinating services, managing finances, and, for 13 percent, providing personal care. These responsibilities lasted an average of three and one-half years for a 30-year-old, but extended to more than six years when the caregiver was over age 40.

Working caregivers face the competing demands of child care, providing care to their older loved one, and work-related responsibilities. This results in the need to adjust work schedules, to cut back hours, or to take time off without pay. About 10 percent of working caregivers, most of them women, eventually quit their jobs.

Caregiving is work. Employers can compare caregivers to employees who have second jobs. For many, caregiving is burdensome and creates conflicts with the responsibilities of work.

WORKING WOMEN AS CAREGIVERS

Elaine Brody, of the Philadelphia Geriatric Center studied women caregivers. Those who quit work to provide care were older—usually in their mid-fifties and tended to have less education and lower overall family income.

Women who were professionals, were younger, or had higher overall family income generally had less conflict between work and their caregiving responsibilities. Fewer hours of direct care resulted in a reduction of home-job conflict.

When caregiving responsibilities reached 20 hours a week, Brody found, the worker began to experience a greater conflict between work and caregiving. Caregivers who ultimately quit work provided an average of 38 hours of care per week.

The positive side of caregiving is that it tends to reinforce strong family networks and intergenerational reciprocity. Such widespread caregiving by family members also lessens society's tax burden for formal caregiving services. It is to the mutual benefit of the employer and the employee to work with the responsibilities of caregiving.

Amy Horowitz of the Lighthouse for the Blind reminds us that while work may lessen the time for caregiving, it may provide important relief from the constant care of an older family member. Yet caregiving responsibilities may affect decisions about work and early retirement for about 15 percent of the nation's caregiving work force.

Marjorie Cantor of the Third Age Center at Fordham University studied caregiving spouses. She found that they are often older, with children who have left home. They experience more stress, worry more, and are often in poorer health than other caregivers. This is partly because spouses more often provide personal care as well as assume responsibilities for household management.

About one-half of spousal caregivers are men, who may have had little experience in running a household or with providing personal care. Assuming these new responsibilities often requires a difficult role reversal for husbands. But children, mostly women, experience a great deal of strain in caring for an older relative, partially due to intergenerational differences and the reversal of the parent-child relationship.

All caregivers, regardless of their age, sex, or relationship to the care recipient, feel strain because of their concern for the health and well-being of the recipient. For working caregivers, job performance may be affected by this stress.

Cantor suggests that flexible work schedules and leave time for caregiving may ease the strain and improve performance in the workplace.

CAREGIVERS' PROGRAMS

The first step in the process of fostering an enlightened workplace is to identify those workers who are burdened with caring for an older relative or friend. The Travelers Insurance Companies began with its survey of employees. International Business Machines (IBM) began in 1986 by hiring a consulting firm to conduct a feasibility survey and develop a corporate program for employee-caregivers.

Other employers have approached the problem of parent care in the same way they have addressed child care responsibilities. The difference in approaching these two types of responsibilities may lie in the social nature of the situations. The trials and tribulations of caring for a child are readily discussed with friends and coworkers. But caregiving for an older relative is often an isolated activity carried out in the privacy of the home.

A number of firms have established programs that assist employees with balancing the burden of care with the responsibilities of work. These plans usually involve providing employees with caregiving information, support, and benefits. Much of the frustration of caregiving derives from feelings of helplessness, burden, and isolation. Providing information about support services is an important first step for employers.

Despite the fact that many services for frail seniors exist in each of our communities, information about such services is often difficult to obtain. Centralizing the information in resource books, an employee assistance office, or, as Travelers did, by holding a caregivers' fair, are a few of the ways for caregiving employees to learn about available community resources.

At the Travelers' fair, 20 community agencies provided information on home and day care, legal and financial help, and coping with stress. Company employees and retirees attended.

Florida Power & Light Company (FPL) has established an eldercare referral network through which the employee assistance program (EAP) provides relief from the stress that often accompanies caregiving. In addition, the EAP works with FPL's Special Consumer Services Department to provide employee-caregivers with up-to-date information about community support services.

FPL also offers employees a tax-free Dependent Care Assistance Benefits program, caregivers fairs, a caregiving video and book resource library and lunch-time seminars.

At IBM, an elder care consultation and referral service has been developed as a source of information for caregiving employees. In addition to information about community resources, the service offers information on specific caregiving issues such as Alzheimer's disease, legal guardianship, and elder care.

American Express Company introduced a benefit that allows employees to purchase long-term care insurance at a group rate. They also offer a dependent care account, an employee assistance program (EAP), and are in the process of developing several initiatives to ease financial access to community resources.

Blue Cross and Blue Shield of Indiana, with a work force that is about 80 percent women, offers "flex-time," described as the opportunity to work 7.5 hours between 6 a.m. and 8:30 p.m.

People's Bank offers a lunch-time forum on elder care, sponsored by the University of Bridgeport, access to a "hotline" at the University of Bridgeport campus, and the availability of outside contract counselors for their employees. People's is also offering leave of absence benefits to employee caregivers and plans to offer retirement seminars.

Stride Rite, a shoe manufacturer based in Cambridge, MA, appears to be a real trend-setter in the pioneering work of elder care. The company offers an eight-week paid maternity leave and an 18-week family leave.

In surveying employees on elder care responsibilities, Stride Rite found that one in four were providing care to an elderly relative. Another 13 percent expected to take on caregiving responsibilities within the next five years. In response, the Stride Rite Children's Center, Lesley College, and Somerville-Cambridge Elder Services worked together to address the needs for affordable, quality care for children and elders. The result: an employer-sponsored, on-site intergenerational day care center.

Ukrops, Inc., a supermarket chain based in Richmond, VA, provides cash benefits to reimburse employees with elder care expenses.

NCNB, the nation's ninth largest bank, which is based in Charlotte, North Caroline, allows employees at all levels to reduce time and job commitments to care for dependents with out cutting off advancement opportunities. "Select Time" allows caregivers to avoid the negative implication that part-time workers are less than fully committed to their jobs.

AT&T provides unpaid leave up to one year, with a job guarantee, for new parents and for workers with seriously ill dependents.

Eastman Kodak now allows part-time work, job sharing, and informal flextime.

Aetna, Ciby-Geigy, and Johnson and Johnson have provided employee seminars on the "ins" and "outs" of Medicare and other government programs.

Consolidated Edison Co. of New York and Mobile Oil Corporation are providing information to support their employee caregivers.

Southwestern Bell Telephone Co. developed a program kit that includes a 28-minute documentary that provides information about elder care and available resources, such as day care.

Corestates Financial Corporation of Philadelphia has a work force of 8.500. Sixty-five percent are women. The company allows employees to select different program options offered by the Aging and the Workplace Program to suit their corporate and employee needs.

Many firms provide articles on elder care in company newsletters. Others offer their employees information through videotapes. Adding relevant materials in the corporate library is yet another strategy. For the caregiver who does not know where to begin to look for assistance, these activities help to reduce employee stress and improve productivity.

Learning that others have similar responsibilities for older relatives is comforting to the employee who may be providing care in isolation. Creating access to support groups is a role ideally suited to larger employers. The Travelers initiated lunchtime seminars on topics including family decision making, coping with mental changes, and legal considerations. These seminars used an informal discussion format, which encouraged the open expression and sharing of concerns. Weekly support groups, staffed by the employee assistance counselor, allowed caregivers to share problems and solutions. Smaller firms have worked with community resources such as a senior center, synagogue, or church to establish similar support groups. Providing such support can reduce anxiety and tension and restore what may be a caregiver's most essential asset: a sense of humor.

Adjusting the benefits package is a special way in which the employer can ease the burden of balancing work and caregiving responsibilities. The Travelers instituted flexible work time in 1984 to assist employees in fulfilling their caregiving commitments. Allowing for personal leave days instead of sick days or providing for unpaid personal leave time are other ways employers can assist their employees. Other benefits might include reimbursed day care, meals with care recipients in the staff cafeteria, work-at-home assignments, and other programs that help employees to more comfortably manage responsibilities of both care and work.

STATE GOVERNMENT PLANS

State governments also are involved in addressing family issues of workers. Of 42 states that responded to a 1990 survey, 28 indicated that they had made a special effort to focus on family issues during a legislative session within the past two years. Twenty-five states focused on legislation related to elderly caregiving. Thirteen introduced family leave legislation, although only three states passed it.

Connecticut's family policy package provided state employees with 24 weeks of unpaid leave during any two-year period upon the birth or adoption of a child or in the event that serious health needs of a child or elderly parent arise.

California established a joint legislative task force on the changing family which emphasized themes including parenting, family economics, aging, and family and the workplace issues.

Massachusetts' initiative on family caregivers insurance requires all employers to offer up to 26 weeks of leave with job security guaranteed. Insurance would replace 66 percent of caregivers' income, up to $237.60 weekly. Employers and employees contribute equally to the insurance fund.

Florida's Department of Administration in 1990 conducted a Caregiver's Fair for state employees in the Tallahassee area as a part of the Family Supportive Work Program Pilot Project (FSWPPP). Representatives of 26 organizations providing services to the elderly participated.

CONGRESS ACTS

After much debate, the Congress in 1993 approved a family leave. The new law requires employers to give up to 12 weeks of unpaid, job-protected leave for the birth, adoption, or serious illness of a child, spouse, or parent.

Knowledge of how employers can assist employees during the caregiving years is just developing. As experience is gained, firms should be encouraged to share methods that improve employee productivity. As one corporate chief executive officer put it, "It's a matter of dollars and sense."

If you are a working caregiver, contact your employer's director of employee benefits to see whether special assistance or counseling is available to you. If you are an employee benefits manager, think about how you may incorporate special programs or assistance into your employee benefits plan.

The Employee Benefit Research Institute (EBRI), at 2121 K St., NW, Suite 600, Washington, DC 20037-1896, publishes information on employee benefit programs, including employee assistance programs and dependent care. Write, or call (202) 775-6315, to inquire about information on programs directed toward caregivers. For a list of EBRI publications, call (410) 516-6946.

References

Cantor, M.D. (1983). "Strain among Caregivers: A Study of Experience in the United States." *The Gerontologist* 23 (6), 597–604.

Horowitz, A. (1985). "Family Caregiving to the Frail Elderly." *Annual Review in Gerontology and Geriatrics*, 194-246.

Piktialis, D.S. (1990). "Employers and Elder Care: A Model Corporate Program." *Pride Institute Journal of Long-Term Home Health Care* 9 (1), 26-31.

Project Share. *Family Caregiving Project.* Rockville, MD: Project Share, Berul Associates, Ltd. (HHS Contract-100-83-0080), 1987.

Stone, R.I., G.L. Cafferata and J. Sangl (1987). "Caregivers of the Frail Elderly: A National Profile." *The Gerontologist* 27 (5), 616–626.

Stone, R.I. & P. Kemper (1989). "Spouses and Children of Disabled Elders: How Large a Constituency for Long-Term Care Reform?" *The Milbank Quarterly* 67 (3–4), 485-506.

The Travelers Employee Caregiver Survey: *A Survey on Caregiving Responsibilities of Travelers Employees for Older Americans.* Hartford, CT: The Travelers Insurance Companies, 1985.

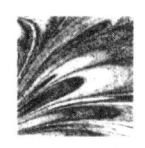

One Corporation's Response to the Needs of Caregivers

Many utilities, including electric, gas, and water, have special consumer programs that may lighten the burden of the caregiver. The following programs, offered by Florida Power & Light Company, are just one utility's response to their customers and employees.

The 62Plus Payment Plan

Created because many seniors and retirees are on fixed incomes, this program moves the payment due date for qualified customers so that it is close to the day that their monthly pension or Social Security checks arrive.

Double Notice Protection Plan

Many people forget to pay their bills or unable to pay them on time, because they are ill or traveling. To help prevent electricity from being disconnected, FPL offers this plan, in which caregivers, family members or neighbors are named to receive a copy of any final notice issued by the utility. This protects the customer from possible disconnection of service because his or her bill mistakenly went unpaid.

Life-Sustaining Medical Equipment Program

This program is for customers who depend on medical equipment prescribed by a doctor and whose life would be in danger without it. Through this program, FPL lets customers know when electric power will be turned off for special repairs. It also makes certain that customers are called if there is a weather emergency that might interrupt electric power.

Assist Program

Serious financial problems can hit any family or individual. The loss of a job, sickness, or an accident can make it difficult for a family to pay its bills. FPL's Assist Program helps customers reach the social service organization(s) that can offer the type of assistance they need. This could include "energy assistance," which helps in paying electric bills. This assistance is made possible in part through donations from customers and FPL corporate contributions through the Care to Share program.

If you would like information about these and other FPL special consumer services, call 1-800-DIAL FPL (1-800-342-5375). Hearing or speech-impaired customers with TT (TTY-TDD) systems may call 1-800-432-6554.

14

Advocating for the Care Recipient

Creston Nelson-Morrill

When I was a little girl, my mother would tell me stories from her childhood in Oklahoma. One of those stories was about an aged Indian chief who would make a daily pilgrimage from a nearby reservation to the Red Rock post office, where my grandfather served as postmaster. My mother, who frequently accompanied my grandfather to work, relished the old chief's visits. The chief was a kind, proud man. Every morning he would ask my grandfather whether any mail had arrived for him. No mail ever came.

The chief's wistful response was always the same:

"All friends dead," he would say, shaking his head. "All friends dead."

Hearing that story as a child, I never dreamed that my mother, too, would one day live in isolation, cut off by illness from her few remaining friends and family members. I never imagined that the day would come when I would be my mother's lifeline to the world.

I am a caregiver.

I am 39 years old. My mother is 88. I am a wife, the mother of three young children, and the president of an allegedly for-profit business. I seriously contemplated committing a capital offense against the last person who asked me what my hobbies are. Does sleeping qualify as a hobby?

In my four years as caregiver to a nursing home resident, in my previous four-and-a-half years as an in-home caregiver, and, even earlier, in my five years as an observer of my mother's caregiving for my late father, I have learned a great deal.

I have learned that no matter how well others think that I am caring for my mother, it will never be good enough for me.

I have learned that there is no such thing as an "easy" caregiving situation; yet I realize that there are many caregivers who have problems far more difficult than mine.

I have learned that the health care and social services "systems" are in reality non-systems, and that anything short of an extraordinarily organized approach to either of them will be frustrating at best—and fatal at worst.

I have learned that no amount of counseling or professional know-how will make the quilt go away when someone you love outlives his or her ability to function.

One of my greatest frustrations as a caregiver has been my inability to translate my professional knowledge of the health care and social services systems into appropriate assistance and care for my mother and me.

I have found that inappropriate referrals are the rule, not the exception. Beware the physician with good intentions but little practical knowledge of case management for older persons.

I have found that front-line workers in the social services system, many of whom are paid at or only slightly above the minimum wage, may not be extraordinarily motivated to help you. I have learned never to expect to hit pay dirt with a single call, even if the organization I am calling should, logically, be able to give me the information and/or support that I need.

Finally, I have found that if the offering of a particular service is logical and would dramatically ease the burden of the caregiver, that service is probably offered only through an under-funded social services organization, whose limited resources are stretched across a number of essential program areas. If a service is offered, do not give up until you find it. If it is not offered, find out why and take your case to a city or county commissioner and/or your state representative or senator.

The bottom line: if you do not have a core of inner strength, do not become a caregiver. Do something easier, like leading a herd of buffalo through a mine field.

After years of blundering through the system, I have concluded that the single best source of information on services available to the elderly and their caregivers in Florida are the local *Elder Helplines*. The *HelpLines* are run by providers under contract with area agencies on aging (AAAs) in each of 11 program service areas. AAA programs in some areas of the state are more innovatively and enthusiastically run than others; all operate on a shoestring budget. Each should be able to provide a resource directory identifying services available in the area to older persons and their caregivers. A complete listing of the *Elder Helpline*s, the AAAs, and area aging program offices is included in Chapter 16.

Before you toss this book aside and make a bee-line for the nearest telephone, some words of advice.

Conduct your own needs assessment. What is the care recipient's and your own physical and mental condition? What are your areas of most critical need? What factors are at work in the care recipient's overall wellness/illness profile (health problems, losses, role changes, family interactions, depression, and/or emotional difficulties)? Write it down.

Know generally what services are available. It will be to your benefit if the person you reach for assistance can spend his or her time on the telephone with you discussing practical alternatives rather than providing basic definitions of services.

If possible, start your quest for information early in the day, when you and the person you reach for assistance are fresh. Never call a state government or government-sponsored office after 4:30 p.m. The person you reach has likely had a rough day and is looking forward to going home or to a second job. It will show.

Be prepared to deal with disinterest or ignorance of the subject matter on the part of the first three persons you reach. If you get the assistance you need on your first try, you should feel triply blessed. Never give up. If you are not getting the help you need, ask to speak to another counselor, to the assistant director, or to the program director. If there are no signs of intelligent life at the program office in your county, try a program in a nearby county. If all else fails, call Tallahassee and make anyone who will listen aware of your difficulties.

Services and Service Providers

ADULT CONGREGATE LIVING FACILITIES (ACLFS)

There are more than 1,600 licensed adult congregate living facilities (ACLFs) in Florida. ACLFs offer independent living with central dining, transportation, and social and recreational programs. In most facilities, residents must be continent and able to function independently.

In 1993, 13 ACLFs had been licensed to provide *extended congregate care,* which allows residents to "age in place," unless the patient's condition requires 24-hour skilled nursing care. Only when it has been determined that a patient requires 24-hour skilled care will he or she be moved from the ACLF, which is considered community-based care, into a nursing home, which provides institutional care.

ACLFs are licensed by the Agency for Health Care Administration (AHCA) under one of three standards:

A *provisional* license is granted for a period of three to six months when there is a change in facility ownership. Occasionally, a start-up facility will receive a provisional license when the AHCA determines that there may be a need for additional review.

A *conditional* license is issued when the AHCA determines that deficiencies exist with a facility licensure application or with the facility, itself.

A *standard* license is issued biennially to facilities meeting all state licensure requirements.

In considering placement in an ACLF, you and/or the care recipient should ask the following questions:

- What is the ACLF's licensure status?
- If you will be paying on a monthly basis, what does the monthly fee include? Are there add-ons (i.e. laundry charges, pharmacy, television, telephone, etc.)? If a deposit is required, is it fully refundable?
- Is transportation available to stores, places of worship, doctors' offices, etc.? Is there a charge for this service? How frequently and flexibly is it available?
- What are the ACLF's policies regarding bringing in the care recipient's own furniture, smoking, visitors, and pets?
- Is there adequate security for personal belongings?

The AHCA makes available to the public a current printout of all ACLFs licensed in Florida. The printout includes the facility name and address, its licensure status, and the facility size. There is a $20 charge for the printout. The Office of Health Facility Regulation is located at 2727 Mahan Drive, Tallahassee, FL, 32308, telephone (904) 487-2515.

ADULT CAY CARE

Adult day care centers provide comprehensive services ranging from health assessment and care to social programs for older persons in need of assistance with activities of daily living but not around-the-clock care. Many centers are supported by state funds, but they may also be operated by hospitals, nursing homes, local government, or religious, civic, or other groups. Easter Seal operates a number of programs in Florida for developmentally disabled and older persons.

In Florida, adult day care centers serving three or more adults unrelated to the operator are licensed by the AHCA. A printout of all adult day care centers licensed by the state is available from the AHCA for $10.

CAREGIVER SUPPORT PROGRAMS

The forgotten person in the caregiving picture is often the most important one: the caregiver.

There is increasing recognition of the emotional and physical toll of caregiving, even on a young and healthy individual, who can make caregiving his or her full-time vocation. Some members of the corporate community are beginning to target working caregivers for special assistance. Social service organizations, health care providers, and religious groups, which used to view the care recipient as the center of the caregiving universe, are increasingly turning their attention to the health and psychological well-being of the caregiver.

Support groups may be run through county school system adult education programs, through hospital community education programs, or by social service organizations. Even if the thought of participating in a support group ranks last on your list of priorities, make a commitment to attend just once. If you are not the type to bare your soul in public, listen to what others have to say. In the unlikely event you are pressed to comment, simply say, "I came to listen and learn."

The question you should ask when you contact the *Elder Helpline* is:

Is there a caregiver's support group or network in my area, and whom can I call for information?

CARRIER WATCH

This is not available in all areas. A sticker placed inside the care recipient's mailbox alerts the postal carrier that an older person lives at that address. Should mail begin to accumulate, the postal carrier will notify the local sheriff's department if he or she has not been previously notified of the resident's absence.

CONGREGATE MEALS

Provided through the Older Americans Act nutrition program, the congregate meals programs provide meals, recreation, and education at one or more sites in a given county. Transportation generally is available to the meal site.

CONTINUING CARE RETIREMENT COMMUNITIES

More than 100,000 Americans reside in continuing care retirement communities (CCRCs). In Florida there were 76 CCRCs in 1993, down from 80-plus in 1990. All are licensed by the Department of Insurance.

CCRCs typically provide independent and assisted living arrangements; many offer intermediate care and skilled nursing facilities. They may be Medicare and/or Medicaid certified.

An insurance department Consumers Guide to Continuing Care Retirement Communities cautions that CCRCs are not the answer to long-term care needs for many seniors. Entrance fees typically range from $15,000 to more than $200,000. Monthly fees range from $250 to $1,500 or more. Independent and assisted living residents live in private apartments, have access to dining rooms for meals, and may participate in a number of social activities.

One of the primary attractions of CCRCs is the promise of financial security and peace of mind. But the Department of Insurance reports that about 40 CCRCs in 10 states have declared bankruptcy since 1975. Therefore, it is important that you choose your CCRC carefully.

Contact your local Department of Insurance consumer service office. A listing of these offices is included in Chapter 16. If there is not one in your area, contact the state office that handles CCRC licensure: Bureau of Specialty Insurers, Florida Department of Insurance, 200 E. Gaines St., Larson Building, Tallahassee, FL 32399-0300, or telephone (904) 922-3144. In addition to the Consumers Guide, the bureau can provide a list of licensed CCRCs, which includes information on admission charges and services.

Spend time at the facility. Make unannounced visits. Talk to residents and find out what they think about the facility. If possible, spend a weekend at the CCRC and participate in some of its planned activities.

Go with your gut. If something does not seem right, it may not be right. Even if there is not a real problem, your peace of mind should come first and foremost.

FOSTER CARE

The adult foster care program is designed to place older persons in need of a minimum amount of assistance into a family environment. Services, provided on a nonprofit basis, include room, board, personal assistance, general supervision, and health monitoring.

Adult foster homes are licensed by the Department of HRS, Aging and Adult Services office and must pass sanitation and fire safety inspections prior to licensure. In addition, references are obtained for all applicants. Both the applicants and household members aged 18 and older must undergo Florida Department of Law Enforcement background checks and abuse registry clearances. Procedures are in place to ensure that all applicants comply with these requirements.

Counselors provide follow-up services to clients on at least a quarterly basis. Clients pay for the cost of their care with their income, usually Social Security, Supplemental Security Income, or, if their income falls below the recognized cost of care ($575 per month in 1993), Optional State Supplementation.

As of July 1993, there were 584 adult foster homes. No more than three nonrelatives who are aged or disabled adults reside in each home. Effective Jan. 1, 1994, the name of the program will change to adult family care and the maximum number of nonrelative residents will increase from three to five.

For additional information on adult foster care, contact the Department of HRS, Adult Foster Home Program, 1317 Winewood Blvd., Tallahassee, FL 32399-0700, telephone (904) 488-2881.

FRIENDLY VISITORS

Friendly visitors are part of an informal network of civic or religious group volunteers who regularly visit older persons. They provide companionship and can assist the care recipient with simple tasks such as reading, writing letters, or running errands.

Contact churches, synagogues, or civic organizations in your area to see whether they have programs.

HEALTH CARE PROFESSIONALS

In Florida, all health care professionals are licensed by the Department of Professional Regulation. Those regulated by the department include: acupuncturists, chiropractors, clinical social workers, dentists, dietitians, hearing aid specialists, marriage and family therapists, massage therapists, naturopaths, nurses, nursing home administrators, opticians, optometrists, osteopaths, pharmacists, physical therapists, physicians, podiatrists, psychiatrists, respiratory therapists, and speech pathologists and audiologists. The Department also licenses funeral directors.

In selecting a health care professional, first and foremost, find someone you and the care recipient are comfortable with. You may not always agree with the care recipient's personal prejudices. But if the care recipient does not trust anyone with a beard, find a health care professional without facial hair. If the care recipient has little faith in women health care professionals, do not press the issue.

Ask for referrals from friends and family members, but bear in mind that the care recipient's special needs may differ from theirs. Check the Yellow Pages or contact the county medical society in the county in which you reside for a list of physicians specializing in geriatric medicine.

Assess the health care professional's style. The physician who seldom keeps you waiting may be the one who will be so interested in keeping on top of his or her schedule that he or she may not have time to get to know you. On the other hand, the physician who keeps you waiting may be the one who will spend extra time with you when you or the care recipient need it.

Check the health care professional's credentials with the Department of Professional Regulation. The department a toll-free number you can call to determine whether a health care professional's license is current and in good standing: (800) 342-7940. While the department cannot comment on cases against a health care professional in which "probable cause" has not yet been determined, you can generally judge from the response whether a case is pending. If there are no cases filed against the health care professional, you will be told so. If a case is pending, you may be told that "no public information is available" on the individual.

Regulation of health care professionals was slated to be moved to the Agency for Health Care Administration (AHCA), effective July 1, 1994.

HOME HEALTH CARE

Home health agencies provide nursing and rehabilitative services to homebound patients with chronic or temporarily debilitating conditions and to individuals recovering in their own homes from major medical treatment.

Services provided include: nursing services by registered or licensed practical nurses; personal care by home health aides (certified nursing assistants); medical social services; sitter and homemaker services; various forms of therapy, including speech and physical; medical supplies, including surgical dressings and catheters; and durable medical equipment, including walkers, wheelchairs, and hospital beds.

There are strict limits on reimbursement for home health care services under both the federal Medicare and state Medicaid programs. The cost of ongoing care by a home health aide or attendance by a sitter deemed not to be medically necessary will be borne by the care recipient or his or her caregiver. Around-the-clock care provided by certified nursing assistants (CNAs) can cost more than $1,500 per week.

There are close to 1,200 agencies in Florida, alone. While Florida home health agencies are licensed by the AHCA and resurveyed on a yearly basis, there is no rating system of ongoing agency performance. State law restricts the activities of the various types of professionals and nonprofessionals employed by home health agencies and establishes minimum standards for case management. Agencies are required to run criminal history and abuse-related background checks on all employees at the time they are hired.

Questions to ask when you contact a home health agency include:

- What is the agency's license number? In Florida, a call to the AHCA, Office of Health Facility Regulation can provide quick verification of an agency's licensure status.
- What services are available?
- What is the hourly charge for a particular service? How will you be billed (i.e., weekly, monthly)? Can someone at the agency assist you with the determination of whether the care recipient may be eligible for care through his or her private insurance, Medicare, or Medicaid?
- Does the home health agency have a patient needs assessment process? If so, what does it entail and who performs the assessment?
- Does the home health agency conduct supervisory visits to the home and, if so, how frequently and by whom?

- Ask the name of the home health agency's medical director and director of nursing. In Florida, you can verify the licensure status of each of these individuals and check for administrative charges filed against them by contacting the Department of Professional Regulation.
- If the care recipient will require regular care, can the agency assure some continuity of care through avoiding constant turnover of personnel?
- Does the home health agency offer its employees initial orientation or continuing education programs?
- Does the agency carry liability insurance and workers' compensation coverage for all employees?

Answers to these question should be in writing on company letterhead, dated and signed by the supervisor.

An area of concern, regardless of whether you go through an agency or attempt to hire home help directly, lies in the area of CNA certification. Unlike most health professionals in Florida, CNAs are not licensed by the Department of Professional Regulation. Instead, they are certified by the Department of Education.

There is no ongoing regulation of CNAs working in the home once they are certified—and certification is for life. There is no requirement for continuing education. Certification involves taking a $20, 80-question exam. Those applying for certification must have completed 100 credit hours of course work or be able to show proof of previous experience as a home health aide.

If you decide to hire a CNA independently of an agency, you should request an abuse registry background check form from the background screener at your district Department of HRS office. Ask any potential employee to fill out the form and sign it, giving permission for HRS to release information to you. Then return the form to the district background screener.

A list of the 11 HRS Aging and Adult Services area background screeners is included in Chapter 16.

You may also want to run a background check through the Florida Department of Law Enforcement. Requests should include the potential employee's name, sex, race, date of birth, and Social Security number and should be addressed to the Florida Department of Law Enforcement,

Name Search Unit, P.O. Box 1489, Tallahassee, FL 32302. There is a $15 charge for this service.

HOMEMAKER SERVICES

Homemaker services provide assistance with light housekeeping, laundry, grocery shopping, and household management.

In Florida, homemakers, sitters, and companions who provide home health services must register with the AHCA. Certificates of registration are valid for one year. The homemaker, sitter, or companion must include in any advertising his or her registration number.

You should conduct a criminal and abuse history background check of potential employees and determine whether they are properly registered with the state.

HOSPICE

Hospice is intended to provide physical, emotional, social, and spiritual care to persons who have been diagnosed with a life-limiting illness or condition and who have a prognosis of less than one year of life. They also provide support to caregivers during the care recipient's illness and the caregiver's period of bereavement.

Hospice programs are medically directed, nurse-coordinated programs providing care to the terminally ill and their families. Plans of care for individual patients are delivered by an interdisciplinary team including a medical doctor, a registered nurse, a social worker, a clergy person or counselor, and hospice-certified volunteers.

Florida's Medicaid and Medicare hospice programs include four levels of care: routine home care, provided on a regular basis at home; continuous home care, providing 24-hour care; inpatient respite care, to provide caregivers a break from the stress of caring for a terminally ill patient; and general inpatient services, provided in a nursing home, hospital, or hospice.

Several national studies have concluded that hospice programs not only improve quality of life but can actually save money for care recipients and the health care system as a whole. One study found that while non-hospice patients spend an average of 6.7 days in the hospital during their last two weeks of life, hospice patients spend an average of 1.6 days in the hospital.

The Big Bend Hospice, Inc., located in Tallahassee, offers the following explanation of what a hospice is and is not:

Advocating

Hospice generally is not a place, a hospital. It is a way of providing care wherever the patient is, at home or in an institution.

Hospice is not a place to send people to die. Rather, hospice is a way of helping people to live out the remainder of their lives with as much comfort and dignity as possible.

Hospice is not a "death bed" service for people. It is a comprehensive care program for patients and families that emphasizes quality of life and is most effective during the final six months of life expectancy.

Hospice is not a place to send dying patients so they will not know what is happening to them. Hospice is a care system based on the right of people to know accurately and honestly what is happening to them so that they can choose how they want to spend their precious remaining amount of time in the most purposeful and meaningful way, consistent with their wishes and needs.

Hospice is not a place to send dying patients to get them out of the way. It is a care system committed to the provision of support to patients and families to help families deal with the stress of caring for a dying family member, and to assist families through the time of bereavement.

Hospice is not for everyone. It is a system of care chosen by some patients and families because it helps them meet their own goals and is consistent with their values.

Hospice is not just for cancer patients. It is available to patients of any age, race, sex, or religion who have a disease in its final stages.

Hospice is not a resignation to hopelessness and helplessness. It is a way to deal realistically and humanely with one of the great challenges of human life, and offers new perspectives on hope and help to patients and their family members.

Hospice is not a substitute for family. Hospice is a family-oriented program that helps families care for their loved ones in their own homes and provides institutional back-up as needed.

Hospice is not expensive, but, rather, emphasizes cost savings by keeping the patient at home, in the family's care. Medicare, Medicaid, and many private insurance companies provide reimbursement for services. No patient is ever denied care because of his or her inability to pay.

Florida was the first state to establish licensure for hospices. The first hospice, Methodist Hospice in Jacksonville, was licensed in 1980. Hospice services now are provided in all 67 Florida counties. To locate the hospice program nearest you, contact the local *Elder Helpline* or check your Yellow Pages.

MEALS ON WHEELS

Older persons who have been assessed as homebound are eligible to receive Meals on Wheels in their homes if they are unable to prepare their own meals. As funding for the program is limited, preference is given to older persons with the greatest need. The service is available on a long- or short-term basis.

Meals are delivered to the homebound weekdays at around noon. They are nutritionally balanced, delivering about two-thirds of the Recommended Dietary Allowance.

NURSE REGISTRIES

Nurse registries are employment agencies that play "matchmaker" between registered nurses, licensed practical nurses and, in some cases, certified nursing assistants and those in need of care. Unlike home health agencies, which employ the health care providers, nurse registries serve as a placement service. Once a provider is placed in your employ, you have the responsibility of supervising care and of calculating and collecting withholding from wages for deposit with the federal government.

Nurse registries' services generally are not covered by private insurance or government programs, meaning that you likely will have to bear the full cost out of pocket. There are about 50 nurse registries in Florida. Check the Yellow Pages in your local telephone directory to determine whether there are any in your area.

NURSING HOMES

Nursing home care is the most intensive form of care in the continuum of long-term care for the elderly. For some elderly persons, nursing home care temporarily follows a severe illness, while others may stay for extended periods of time. Other elderly persons live in nursing homes until they die.

Nursing homes provide a wide range of rehabilitative, restorative, and other services, including speech, physical, and occupational therapy; pharmaceutical services; dietary services; laboratory and radiology services; and mental health services.

The American Association of Retired Persons (AARP) contends that nursing homes are intended only for those who are seriously ill—not for people who feel they have no other options.

Nationwide, there are more than 20,000 nursing homes. Together, they serve about 5 percent of the older population. AARP reports that each of us has a 25 percent chance of needing nursing home care at some point in our lives. The likelihood of nursing home placement is higher for older persons residing in areas with colder climates, for those with incomes below the federal poverty level, and for those in need of assistance in basic daily activities such as eating, bathing, and dressing.

In Florida, the number of licensed nursing home beds as of March 1993 was 72,166, up from 29,400 in 1975. Florida's bed-to-population ratio is 34.8 beds per 1,000 persons aged 65 or older, the lowest in the nation. Some states have 85 or more beds per 1,000 older persons.

Just over 2.5 percent of Floridians aged 65 or older live in nursing homes. About 12.5 percent of Floridians over age 85 live in nursing homes.

Florida nursing homes generally provide any of three levels of care. A *skilled nursing facility* provides complex health care services on a 24-hour basis under the supervision of technically or professionally trained personnel. *Intermediate level I* facilities provide care to patients in need of health care services on a daily basis who are mildly incapacitated and need constant supervision to prevent deterioration and disability. *Intermediate level II* facilities serve those who are mildly incapacitated or ill and require health care services on a daily basis. The AHCA reports that few nursing homes are licensed to provide level II care.

The AHCA reviews nursing homes at least once annually and assigns one of three ratings: facilities assigned a *superior* rating exceed all qualifications established by the department; facilities assigned a *standard* rating meet all of those qualifications; and facilities given a *conditional* rating failed to meet the department's minimum standards.

In Florida, the AHCA Office of Health Facilities Regulation, 2727 Mahan Drive, Tallahassee, FL 32308, publishes an annual directory of all nursing homes. Facilities are listed by county, and information provided includes facility name and address, Medicaid and Medicare certification status, number of licensed beds, and rating. There is a $10 charge for the publication.

Factors to consider when choosing a nursing home include:

- What rating has the facility been assigned by HRS? If it has not received a superior or average rating, what deficiencies were noted by the Department in withholding superior status?
- What is the staff to patient ratio? How long has the nursing director worked at the facility? Is there a high staff turnover rate?

- Is the facility clean and odor free? If there is no odor, is it because of superior attention to cleanliness or the absence of incontinent individuals? Some nursing homes will not accept incontinent individuals.
- Are residents given privacy during treatment and care of personal needs? Do residents receive daily personal hygiene needed to assure cleanliness, good skin care, grooming, and oral hygiene? Are residents encouraged to take care of their self-care needs? Are residents free from bedsores?
- Are residents who have problems with bowel and bladder control provided with care necessary to encourage self-control, including frequent toileting and opportunities for rehabilitative training? Are residents afforded rehabilitative nursing care to promote maximum physical functioning to prevent the loss of the ability to walk or move freely?
- Are residents who need assistance in eating or drinking provided prompt assistance?
- Are drugs administered in accordance with the written order of the resident's attending physician?
- Are services provided to meet the residents' social and emotional needs? Does the facility have an ongoing program of meaningful activities based on identified needs and interests of each resident? Is that program designed to promote opportunities for engaging in normal pursuits, including the religious activities of the resident's choice, if any?
- Does the facility develop and implement a written health care plan for each resident according to the instructions of the resident's attending physician and family members? If so, who develops the plan?
- Does the nursing home follow isolation techniques to prevent the spread of infection?
- Is food stored, refrigerated, prepared, distributed, and served under sanitary conditions? Is the food appetizing and well-prepared?

Chapter 11 looks more closely at the nursing home decision and factors the caregiver should take into consideration when selecting a facility.

PERSONAL EMERGENCY RESPONSE SYSTEM

This service is not available in all areas. It provides equipment to monitor the safety of older persons in their own homes through signals that are electronically transmitted over the telephone. In some areas, the older person wears a transmitter "necklace," which he or she can activate should the need for medical assistance arise. The older person's medical records are on file with the monitoring organization so that a quick and appropriate response to a medical emergency is facilitated.

PROFESSIONAL CARE MANAGEMENT

Professional care managers offer professional assistance to assess an individual's need for long-term care and then locate, arrange, and monitor those services. Care managers can coordinate community health and social services. Professional care management may be appropriate if the older person needs the services of a number of different providers or if the would-be caregiver does not live in the area and is unfamiliar with local services.

The National Association of Professional Geriatric Care Managers (NAPGCM) provides a list of professionals across the country who may be able to assist you. The organization is located at 655 Alvernon Way, Suite 108, Tucson, AZ, 85711, or telephone (602) 881-8008. The National Association of Area Agencies on Aging, 600 Maryland Ave., SW, West Wing, Washington, DC 20024, publishes a voluntary standard for professional geriatric care managers.

The American Association of Retired Persons (AARP) advises that you consider the following when choosing a professional care manager:

- What are the care manager's qualifications? If he or she represents him- or herself to be a licensed professional, check to verify licensure status. In addition to regulating a wide range of health care providers, the Department of Professional Regulation also licenses accountants. Determine in advance the process for lodging complaints about the care or the care manager.
- Will the care manager work to determine eligibility for publicly funded programs through Medicare or Medicaid? How knowledgeable is he or she in these areas? Bear in mind that state Medicaid regulations vary significantly from one state to another.
- Will the care manager make a home visit as part of the comprehensive assessment of the care recipient's needs? Will contact with

family members and the care recipient's physician be a part of the comprehensive assessment?

Additional information on professional care management is included in Chapter 4.

RESPITE CARE
Respite care is provided in the home to temporarily relieve the primary caregiver of the responsibility associated with daily full-time care. The service generally is available through the *Elder Helpline* provider agency and through religious and community service organizations.

SENIOR CENTERS
There are a number of senior centers in Florida where older persons may come for meals, social interaction, continuing education opportunities, counseling, or health assessment/wellness programs. Senior centers generally are locally funded and individual programs vary substantially from one center to the next. Some provide transportation to and from the center on a daily basis.

Contact your local *Elder Helpline* to find out if there is a senior center close to you. Contact the center directly for information on activities and programs.

Navigating the System

Creston Nelson-Morrill

There is no long-term care system. Since 1945, life expectancy has increased by 20 years, but we haven't adjusted societally. We leave older people and their caregivers to face a black hole.—E. Bentley Lipscomb, Secretary, Florida Department of Elder Affairs

There's no question that Florida is unique in the nation. With its large aging population, Florida finds itself in 1993 where other states won't be for 20 years. Four Florida counties each account for more spending on long-term care than some states do.

Despite the birth of a new Department of Elder Affairs (DOEA) in October 1991, there still is no single state agency coordinating elder care services. No fewer than 15 state agencies oversee programs that serve the elderly and funding is, by all accounts, insufficient to meet the need. "We have encouraged people to come to Florida after their retirement," Lipscomb says, "but adequate services are lacking."

A May 1993 *Dialogue on Long-Term Care,* sponsored by the DOEA Advisory Council, brought to the table representatives of key state agencies and service providers. Several themes emerged:

- Parts of a system are in place, and services are being provided, but there is no planned, cohesive, integrated long-term care system in Florida. Unless a plan is developed, Florida will not be well-positioned to implement state responsibilities that may be part of national health care reform and will face massive long-term care expenditures.

- Florida's current system has an institutional bias that needs to be balanced with a greater focus on home- and community-based services.
- The geriatric curriculum in Florida medical schools is inadequate to meet the needs of a state with a significant aging population.
- All long-term care providers are experiencing increasing numbers of older, frailer clients in need of more services.
- All long-term care providers are experiencing funding problems. Florida's ability to finance long-term care is in serious jeopardy and its ability to fund long-term care adequately with its current tax base is severely limited.

Rising health care costs, too, have had a severe impact on Florida's elder population. In 1991, the elderly spent more than twice as much, after adjusting for inflation, on out-of-pocket health care costs than they did prior to start-up of the Medicare program. Older persons have the highest out-of-pocket health care costs of any age group, averaging just over 17 percent of income.

Agency for Health Care Administration Director Doug Cook reports that 75 percent of the nursing home population is age 75 or older, with the average annual cost of nursing home care topping $30,000. Statistics compiled by the Health Care Board (HCB) show that 77 percent of nursing home residents are admitted directly from hospitals. Contrary to the public perception that people enter nursing homes and live their until their deaths, the median stay in a nursing home is now 38 days, the HCB data shows.

That points to the changing role of nursing homes as recuperative facilities. With the Medicare program providing economic incentives for shorter hospital stays, sicker, less able persons are being discharged from hospitals. That only serves to complicate the role of the caregiver.

In interviews with caregivers, a common theme emerges: no matter how difficult the challenge—and no matter how superhuman the response—no caregiver believes that he or she is doing enough. We all want to do more. All too often "the system" works against us. All too often we are frustrated in our efforts.

A variety of services are available to older Floridians at all income levels. By learning to work with the agencies that provide services, you will be able to better care for the care recipient and to lighten your load as a caregiver.

The process of recognizing that help is needed, and then finding that help, can be long and frustrating. Services vary from county to county and the mix of agency involvement—particularly the DOEA, the Department of HRS, and the AHCA—is complicated and often confusing. Just remember that you and the person on the other end of the telephone are on the same side. Although it may take some time to get the help you need, there are people willing to guide you.

While the information contained in this chapter will not make that road any shorter, it will give you a starting point for your journey through the service delivery maze.

The Initial Contact

Your local *Elder Helpline* is the first number to call in each of Florida's 67 counties. A complete listing of the local program offices is included in Chapter 16.

The *Elder Helpline* is your entry point to a wide variety of services. You will be referred to other people and organizations, so have paper and pencil ready when you call. Be patient, thorough, and take the time to organize information as you get it so that it will make sense to you later as you attempt to follow up on suggestions.

Make information-gathering calls at a time when you will be able to comfortably spend the time to find people and programs to help you, as the caregiver, and the care recipient. Ask for and write down the names and telephone numbers of the people you speak to so that as you are referred or transferred you will be able to contact them again. Also ask for and write down the names of the documents you will need to have with you if the care recipient needs to prove age or income. These may include the care recipient's birth certificate, his or her Social Security number, income and asset information, information about current living expenses, and bills for medications and physician care.

Be persistent, patient, and polite. Make the person on the other end of the line your ally. Treat the person who answers the telephone as you hope you will be treated.

Since services vary from county to county, the availability of services in a given area may be limited.

Finally, change is in the wind. As we go to press, it appears that legislation will be introduced prior to the 1994 state legislative session transferring many of remaining elder care functions of the Department of HRS' Aging and Adult Services program to the DOEA.

Once You Have Made Contact with the *Elder Helpline*

The person whom you speak with will ask some general questions about your situation and will use that information to let you know what your next step should be. Try to be as specific as possible about your needs. If you have a problem, try to describe it frankly. This will help the person who answers your call to direct it appropriately. If you need only limited assistance or information, you will be referred to a service provider in your area.

If, however, an emergency exists, an Aging and Adult Services case manager may visit you within 24 hours of your call. As you would with any service person who visits your home, ask for identification. The HRS case manager will be comfortable in showing identification to you.

If special assistance is needed, but not on an emergency basis, a case manager may visit within three days of your call. He or she will assess your situation during that visit. The case manager is knowledgeable of community services and will coordinate available resources, including family or church help. If additional assistance is needed, a case manager will continue to work with you to adjust services as your situation changes.

The case manager is the person who will help guide you through the process of determining age and income eligibility, communicate with service providers, and combine the right mixture of services for your needs. As of this writing, services provided directly by HRS fall into three general categories, each of which has different eligibility requirements.

Protective services are provided on an emergency basis if abuse or neglect is occurring. There is no income eligibility requirement for these services.

Supportive services include assistance with housekeeping, meals on wheels, visiting nurses, and many other types of help. Your case manager will work to coordinate a care plan that takes into account the needs of your loved one, your ability to participate as a caregiver, and the availability of services in your community. Income eligibility requirements vary for these services, so rely on your case manager to help you process any necessary paperwork.

Placement services involve moving the person into another environment. These services range from group living facilities to nursing home placement. Again, your case manager will work with you in determining the best solution to your individual caregiving situation. HRS administers programs for older persons at the community level through 11 area offices.

The *Elder Helpline* is Florida's effort to assure quality of life for older persons. It is the key to the information and assistance available in your local community. In every Florida county there is a local telephone number to call for information and assistance. These numbers are included in Chapter 16.

The following state programs are available to assist older Floridians and their caregivers:

ABUSE REGISTRY BACKGROUND SCREENING
In Chapters 4 and 14, we discussed the necessity of conducting Florida Department of Law Enforcement and Central Abuse Registry background checks of potential employees who will be providing care to your loved one.
Abuse registry background screeners are located in each of the 11 Aging and Adult Services service areas. A complete listing is included in Chapter 16.

ADULT CONGREGATE LIVING FACILITY PLACEMENT
Location: Aging and Adult Services
General objectives: To provide an alternative to institutional care for elderly and disabled adults. The program provides room and board with personal care services. HRS clients must be income eligible.
Services: Room, board, and at least one personal care service, such as bathing, dressing, ambulation, and supervision of medication, provided in a congregate situation. The number of residents varies from four to 1,000. For HRS clients, case management, including counseling, escort services, health support, and placement assistance and supervision.
Eligibility: Placement services are open to income-eligible HRS clients only. They must be aged 60 or older or be disabled and over 17 years of age. The must meet income requirements for placement services. Aging and Adult Services counselors must determine that ACLF placement is appropriate.

ADULT FOSTER HOME (EFFECTIVE JAN. 1, 1994 ADULT FAMILY CARE HOME)
Location: Aging and Adult Services
General objectives: To provide a family-like setting, supervision, and maintenance for eligible elderly and disabled adults as an alternative to institutionalization for those who can no longer live independently.
Services: Placement in a family unit where foster sponsors provide maintenance, supervision, and socialization for one to three foster home clients. Case management includes counseling, escort services, health support, and placement assistance and supervision.
Eligibility: The care recipient must be aged 60 or older or be disabled and over age 17. He or she must meet income requirements for placement services. Aging and Adult Services counselors must determine that the client cannot function in his or her own home and that no family member is able or willing to provide care

ALZHEIMER'S DISEASE RESPITE
Location: DOEA
General objectives: To provide respite care so that caregivers may be temporarily relieved of the responsibility associated with daily, full-time care.
Services: Now available in 38 counties, services include in-home, facility-based, emergency, and extended care respite (up to 30 days).
Eligibility: The caregiver must be providing care for a person diagnosed as having probable Alzheimer's disease or another related memory disorder.

ALZHEIMER'S PROJECTS/SERVICES
Location: DOEA
General objectives: To provide respite care, day care, diagnostic services, autopsies, registry, information and referral, and training workshops.
Services: Six components: Alzheimer's Disease Advisory Committee, six memory disorder clinics, seven model Alzheimer's day care programs, Alzheimer's' Disease Research Brain Bank (in cooperation with Mount Sinai Medical Center), Alzheimer's Disease Registry and Information System (in cooperation with the University of South Florida), special projects (funded on an annual basis by the Legislature).
Eligibility: For day care services, the care recipient must have been diagnosed or strongly suspected of having Alzheimer's disease or a related memory disorder, must reside in selected "target" counties, must

be willing to participate in "approved" research projects, must need assistance with activities of daily living and/or need constant supervision for health and safety reasons, and must have a primary caregiver in their residence who needs assistance in caring for the client. For memory disorder clinics, he or she must be suspected of having Alzheimer's Disease or related memory disorders.

COMMUNITY CARE FOR DISABLED ADULTS
Location: Aging and Adult Services
General objectives: To provide supporting services to impaired adults aged 18–59 so that they may remain in the least restrictive environment (i.e., their own home, a relative's home, or a foster/boarding home in the community).
Services: Case management, adult day care, adult day health care, home-delivered meals, homemaker services, personal care, medical transportation, medical supplies and equipment, chore services
Eligibility: The care recipient must be aged 18–59 and be in priority need of services as determined by client assessment. A fee schedule is based on ability to pay, but if income falls below certain levels, services are free.

COMMUNITY CARE FOR THE ELDERLY (CCE) CORE SERVICES
Location: DOEA
General objectives: To provide supportive services to impaired elderly adults to remain in the least restrictive environment (i.e.., their own home, a relative's home, or a foster/boarding home in the community).
Services: Case management, adult day care, health care, home-delivered meals, homemaker services, chore services, medical transportation, respite care, emergency alert response, and personal care.
Eligibility: The care recipient must be aged 60 or older and in priority need of services as determined by client assessment. A fee schedule is based on ability to pay; however,if he or she is receiving Older Americans Act services, SSI, or food stamps or is currently Medicaid-eligible, the means test does not apply.

COMPREHENSIVE ASSESSMENT AND REVIEW FOR LONG-TERM CARE SERVICES (CARES)
Location: Aging and Adult Services
General objectives: To divert elderly adults from nursing home placement to alternative living arrangements and to determine the level

of care appropriate if nursing home care is required.

Services: Preadmission screening for nursing home placement and referrals for services

Eligibility: The care recipient must be 18 years of age or older and be medically in need of services or institutional placement.

DISPLACED HOMEMAKER

Location: Aging and Adult Services

General objectives: To provide supportive services to eligible displaced homemakers in order to promote independence and economic security vital to a productive life.

Services: Counseling, education, employment services, financial management, information and referral, job counseling, job placement, job research, job training, and outreach.

Eligibility: You must be aged 35 or older and have worked in the home providing unpaid household services for family members. You must be unemployed, or must not have achieved economic security based on individual need assessment. You must have had difficulty in securing adequate employment and have been dependent on the income of another family member who no longer supports you or have been dependent on federal assistance. Services are also provided to victims of domestic violence and their dependents.

HOME CARE FOR DISABLED ADULTS

Location: Aging and Adult Services

General objectives: To encourage and support families to care for eligible members at home, as an alternative to institutionalization for disabled adults who can no longer live independently. The care recipient lives with a relative or other caregiver in the community.

Services: Monthly subsidy and supplements are provided to the client's family to care for him or her in the relative's home on a 24-hour basis. Case management.

Eligibility: The care recipient must be aged 18–59 and be financially eligible. He or she must have an approved caregiver and have a priority need for services. The care recipient must meet Medicaid requirements for the lowest level of nursing home care. He or she must be certified as being at risk of institutionalization.

HOME CARE FOR THE ELDERLY (HCE)
Location: Aging and Adult Services
General objectives: To encourage and support families to care for eligible members at home, as an alternative to institutionalization for those who can no longer live independently. The care recipient lives with a relative or other caregiver in the community.
Services: Monthly subsidy and supplements are provided to the client's family to care for him or her in the relative's home on a 24-hour basis. Case management.
Eligibility: The care recipient must be aged 60 or older and be financially eligible. He or she must have an approved caregiver and have a priority need for services. The care recipient must meet Medicaid requirements for the lowest level of nursing home care. He or she must be certified as being at risk of institutionalization.

OLDER AMERICANS ACT (OAA) SERVICES
Location: DOEA
General objectives: To provide planning, advocacy, nutrition, and social services to enable the elderly to live with the maximum possible dignity and independence in the least restrictive environment.
Services: Planning, advocacy, outreach, chore services, companionship, counseling, education, homemaker services, escorting, transportation, legal services, shopping, congregate meals, home-delivered meals, adult day care, employment services, consumer protection, telephone reassurance, information and referral, health support, home health aides, housing improvement, and recreation/social groups.
Eligibility: The care recipient must be aged 60 or older. Their spouses under age 60 may be served meals at congregate sites.

16

Directory of Elder Services and Caregiver Support Organizations

This directory is intended to assist caregivers and their loved ones in finding the services they need. If you discover that a phone number listed here is no longer in service, call your local directory assistance operator (411).

The directory is divided into four parts. First, we have provided telephone numbers for the *Elder Helpline Information & Referral Services* in the 11 Aging and Adult Services planning and service areas (PSAs). This should be the starting point of your quest for services or assistance.

Next, you will find a listing of services and elder care programs in each of the 11 PSAs. These are arranged alphabetically. A map is provided to help determine which PSA you or the care recipient live in. We have included a list of counties that fall within each PSA.

Third, we have included a list of some of the more frequently called numbers for services and programs at the state and national levels. Many of these programs concentrate on research and study of aging issues. Most are not direct providers of services, but they may be able to refer you to local service providers.

Finally, we have included listings for institutions conducting geriatric research.

This chapter provides a sampling of the services and programs available in every area of the state. Most are community-based and are offered by not-for-profit organizations. In addition to the service providers and governmental agencies listed in this chapter, you may also wish to consult your local telephone directory for local chapters of organizations such as mental health associations, the American Cancer Society, the American Heart Association, and Easter Seal.

Elder Helpline Information & Referral Services

Your local *Elder Helpline* is your first and best source of information in every county, it serves as a clearinghouse for elder care information and services.

PSA I
Escambia—(904) 432-1475
Okaloosa—(904) 833-9165
Santa Rosa—(904) 939-0477
Walton—(904) 892-8168

PSA II
Bay—(904) 769-3468
Calhoun—(904) 674-4163
Franklin—(904) 697-3760
Gadsden—(904) 627-2223
Gulf—(904) 229-8466
Holmes—(904) 547-2345
Jackson—(904) 482-5028
Jefferson—(904) 997-3418
Leon—(904) 575-9694
Liberty—(904) 643-5613
Madison—(904) 973-2006
Taylor—(904) 584-4924
Wakulla—(904) 926-7145
Washington—(904) 638-6216

PSA III
Alachua—(904) 336-3822

Bradford—(904) 964-3837
Citrus—(904) 746-1844
Columbia—(904) 755-0235
Dixie—(904) 498-7910
Gilchrist—(904) 463-7681
Hamilton—(904) 792-2136
Hernando—(904) 796-0485
Lafayette—(904) 294-1172
Lake—(904) 326-5304
Levy—(904) 493-1290
Marion—(904) 629-7407
Putnam—(904) 328-2121
Sumter—(904) 793-5234
Suwannee—(904) 364-5673
Union—(904) 496-2922

PSA IV
Baker—(904) 259-2223
Clay—(904) 284-5977
Duval—(904) 798-9503
Flagler—(904) 437-7300
Nassau (Hillard)—(904) 845-3332
Nassau (Fernandina Beach)—(904) 261-0701

St. Johns—(904) 824-1648
Volusia—(800) 544-8127
Volusia (out-of-state)—(904) 253-4700

PSA V
Pasco—(East)—(904) 567-1111
Pasco (Central)—(813) 228-8686
Pasco (West)—(813) 848-5555
Pinellas (813) 531-4664

PSA VI
Hillsborough—(813) 684-6434
Highlands (Avon Park)—(813) 452-1288
Highlands (Lake Placid)—(813) 465-1199
Highlands (Sebring)—(813) 382-1288
Hardee—(813) 773-6880
Manatee—(813) 749-7127
Polk—(800) 533-0741

PSA VII
Brevard—(407) 631-2747
Osceola—(407) 847-4357
Orange—(407) 648-4357
Seminole—(407) 831-4357

PSA VIII
Charlotte—(813) 637-2288
Collier—(813) 774-8443
DeSoto—(813) 494-5965
Glades—(813) 946-1821
Hendry—(813) 983-7088
Lee—(813) 433-3900
Sarasota (North)—(813) 955-2122

Sarasota (Englewood/N. Port)—(813) 475-4056

PSA IX
Indian River—(407) 569-0764
Martin—(407) 283-2242
Okeechobee—(813) 763-9444
Palm Beach—(407) 930-5040
Palm Beach (out-of-state)—(407) 355-4191
St. Lucie—(407) 465-1485

PSA X
Broward—(305) 484-4357

PSA XI
Dade—(305) 358-6060
Monroe—(800) 273-2044

Several Florida state agencies and Elder Helplines *are equipped with Telecommunication Devices for the Deaf (TDDs). The Florida Relay System allows telephone calls to be placed between TDD users and nonusers with the help of specially trained operators translating the calls.*
 1-800-955-8771 (TDD)
 1-800-955-8770 (Voice)

Planning and Service Areas

Area Agency on Aging Headquarters

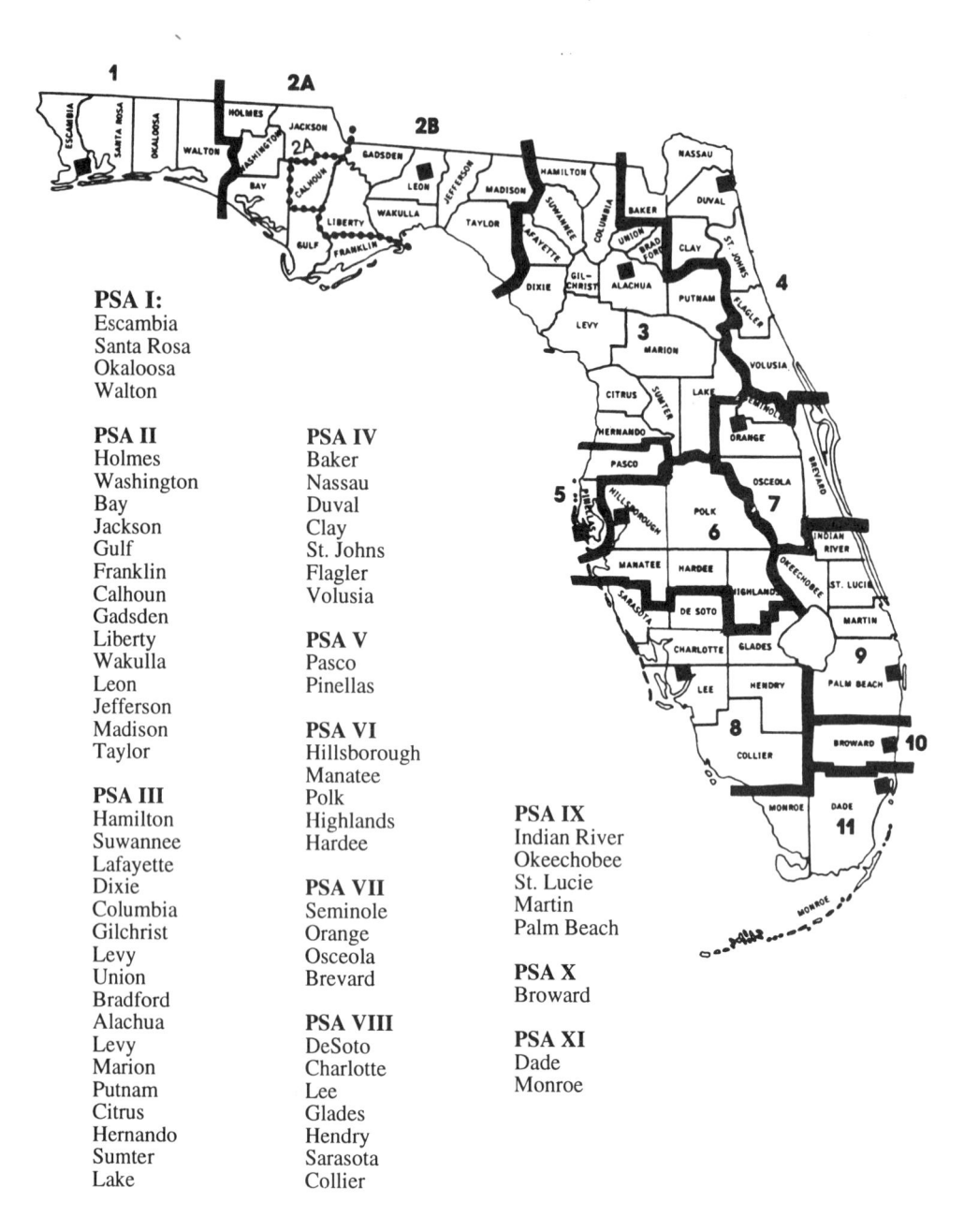

PSA I:
Escambia
Santa Rosa
Okaloosa
Walton

PSA II
Holmes
Washington
Bay
Jackson
Gulf
Franklin
Calhoun
Gadsden
Liberty
Wakulla
Leon
Jefferson
Madison
Taylor

PSA III
Hamilton
Suwannee
Lafayette
Dixie
Columbia
Gilchrist
Levy
Union
Bradford
Alachua
Levy
Marion
Putnam
Citrus
Hernando
Sumter
Lake

PSA IV
Baker
Nassau
Duval
Clay
St. Johns
Flagler
Volusia

PSA V
Pasco
Pinellas

PSA VI
Hillsborough
Manatee
Polk
Highlands
Hardee

PSA VII
Seminole
Orange
Osceola
Brevard

PSA VIII
DeSoto
Charlotte
Lee
Glades
Hendry
Sarasota
Collier

PSA IX
Indian River
Okeechobee
St. Lucie
Martin
Palm Beach

PSA X
Broward

PSA XI
Dade
Monroe

Caregivers Handbook

Local Services Guide
PSA I

Northwest Florida Area Agency on Aging
Dottie Peoples, Executive Director
6706 N. 9th Ave. Bldg. A, Suite 1
Pensacola, FL 32504-7398
(904) 484-5150

Escambia, Santa Rosa, Okaloosa, Walton

Council on Aging Alzheimer's Support Group
105 Santa Rosa Blvd.
Fort Walton Beach, FL 32548
(904) 833-9167

Department of Insurance, Consumer Services
160 Governmental Center, Suite 515
Pensacola, FL 32501
(904) 436-8040

Escambia County Medical Society
Sandra S. DeChamplain, Executive Director
529 Fontaine St.
Pensacola, FL 32503

Hospice of Northwest Florida
P.O. Box 17887
Pensacola, FL 32501
(904) 433-2155

HRS Aging and Adult Services
J.O. Zachow, Program Administrator
P.O. Box 8420
Pensacola, FL 32505-8420
(904) 436-8107

HRS Background Screening Coordinator
160 Governmental Center
P.O. Box 8420, Rm. 410
Pensacola, FL 32505-8420
(904) 436-8135

HRS District Administrator
P.O. Box 8420
Pensacola, FL 32505-8420
(904) 436-8200

HRS Human Services Program Specialist *(Medicaid eligibility determinations)*
160 Governmental Center
P.O. Box 8420
Pensacola, FL 32505-8420
(904) 436-8317

Long-Term Care Ombudsman Council
Donna Brown, Coordinator
160 Government Center
P.O. Box 8420
Pensacola, FL 32505-8420
(904) 436-8243

Mental Health Association Support Group
1995 N. "H" St.
Pensacola, FL 32501
(904) 438-9879

Okaloosa Council on Aging
105 Santa Rosa Blvd.
Fort Walton Beach, FL 32548
(904) 833-9165

Okaloosa County Medical Society
Carolyn Johnson, Executive Secretary
1000 Marwalt Dr.
Fort Walton Beach, FL 32647-6708

Santa Rosa County Medical Society
c/o HCA Santa Rosa Medical Center
P.O. Box 648
Milton, FL 32572

Veterans' Affairs
(Pensacola) (800) 827-1000

Walton County Medical Society
21 College Ave.
DeFuniak Springs, FL 32433

PSA II

Area Agency on Aging, of North Florida, Inc.
Jim Drake, Executive Director
2639 N. Monroe St.,
 Suite 145-B
Tallahassee, FL 32303
(904) 488-0055

Calhoun, Liberty, Wakulla, Leon, Jefferson, Gadsden, Taylor, Washington, Bay, Jackson, Holmes, Gulf, Franklin, Madison

Alzheimer's Association
P.O. Box 1327
Panama City, FL 32402
(904) 763-8258

Alzheimer's Coalition of Tallahassee (ACT)
P.O. Box 3553
Tallahassee, FL 32315
(904) 575-9694

Alzheimer's Disease Initiative
2518 W. Tennessee
Tallahassee, FL 32304
(904) 488-2881

Alzheimer's Resource Center of Tallahassee
1400 N. Monroe St.
P.O. Box 3553
Tallahassee, FL 32303
(904) 561-6869

Apalachee Center for Human Services
Gerontology Program
P.O. Box 1782
Tallahassee, FL 32302
(904) 487-2930

Bay County Senior Center
1116 Frankford Ave.
Panama City, FL 32401
(904) 769-3468

Bays Medical Society
Nancy Canty, Executive Director
P.O. Box 574
Panama City, FL 32402

Big Bend Transit/Medicaid
P.O. Box 1721
Tallahassee, FL 32302
(904) 222-4160

Big Bend Deaf Service Center
2339 Wednesday St.
Tallahassee, FL 32308
(904) 422-3323

Big Bend Hospice
1932 Miccosukee Rd.
Tallahassee, FL 32308
(904) 878-5310

Capital Area Community Action Agency
438 W. Brevard
Tallahassee, FL 32304
(904) 222-2091

Capital Medical Society
Mollie Hill, Executive Director
1204 Miccosukee Rd.
Tallahassee, FL 32308
(904)877-9018

CARES Comprehensive Assessment Program
2639 N. Monroe St., Suite 100 A
Tallahassee, FL 32303
(904) 488-3960

Center for Independent Living of North Florida
1380 Ocala Rd. H-4
Tallahassee, FL 32304
(904) 575-9621

ComFort/Companions for Therapy
2639 N. Monroe St., Suite 145-B
Tallahassee, FL 32303
(904) 488-0055

Community Care for the Elderly/Senior Society Planning Council
2518 W. Tennessee St.
Tallahassee, FL 32304
(904) 575-9694

Dial-A-Ride
555 Appleyard Dr.
Tallahassee, FL 32304
(904) 574-5199

Division of Blind Services
2003 Apalachee Pkwy., #201 Parkway Bldg.
Tallahassee, FL 32399-2950
(904) 488-8400

Elder Care Services
2518 W. Tennessee St.
Tallahassee, FL 32304
(904) 575-9694

Emergency Care Help Organization (ECHO)
702 W. Madison St.
Tallahassee, FL 32304
(904) 224-3246

Emergency Home Energy Assistance/ Senior Planning Society
2518 W. Tennessee St.
Tallahassee, FL 32304
(904) 575-9694

Franklin County Medical Society
Nancy Canty, Executive Director
P.O. Box 574
Panama City, FL 32402

FSU Speech and Hearing Clinic
Department of Communication Disorders
107 RRC
Tallahassee, FL 32306-2007
(904) 644-2238

Gerontology Program/Apalachee Center for Human Services
P.O. Box 1782
Tallahassee, FL 32302
(904) 487-2930

Gulf County Medical Society
Nancy Canty, Executive Director
P.O. Box 574
Panama City, FL 32402

Hearing Aid Referral Program/Elder Services
2518 W. Tennessee St.
Tallahassee, FL 32304
(904) 575-9694

Holmes County Medical Society
Cindy Mathis, Executive Director
P.O. Box 566
Chipley, FL 32428-0566

HRS Aging and Adult Services
Janice Miller, Program Administrator
2639 N. Monroe St., Suite 200-A
Tallahassee, FL 32303
(904) 487-2271

HRS Aging and Adult Services (CARES)
500 W. 11th St.
Panama City, FL 32401
(904) 872-7662

HRS Background Screening Coordinator
2639 N. Monroe St., Suite 200-A
Cedars Executive Center
Tallahassee, FL 32399-2949
(904)488-3960

HRS District Administrator
2639 N. Monroe St., Suite 200-A
Tallahassee, FL 32303
(904) 488-0567

HRS Food Stamp Program
2005 Apalachee Pkwy.
Tallahassee, FL 32301
(904) 488-1182

HRS Human Services Program Specialist *(Medicaid eligibility determinations)*
Suite 200-A
2639 North Monroe St.
Tallahassee, FL 32303
(904) 488-3960

HRS Human Services Program Specialist *(Medicaid eligibility determinations)*
500 West 11th Street
Panama City, FL 32401
(904) 872-7662

Independence for the Blind
1278 Paul Russell Rd.
Tallahassee, FL 32301
(904) 942-3658

Jackson County Medical Society
Cindy Mathis, Executive Director
P.O. Box 566
Chipley, FL 32428-0566

Legal Aid Foundation
301 S. Monroe St., Rm 421
Tallahassee, FL 32301
(904) 222-3004

Leon Association for Retarded Citizens
1572 Capital Circle N.W.
Tallahassee, FL 32303
(904) 575-7521

Lifeline/Tallahassee Memorial Regional Medical Center
(Tallahassee) (904) 681-5315

Life Management Center
525 E. 15th St.
Panama City, FL 32405
(904) 769-9481

Long-Term Care Ombudsman Council
Gwen Schaper, Coordinator
2639 N. Monroe St., Suite 200-A
Tallahassee, FL 32303
(904) 488-9875

Meals on Wheels/Senior Dining
2518 W. Tennessee
Tallahassee, FL 32304
(904) 575-9694

Neighborhood Health Services
548 W. Park Ave.
Tallahassee, FL 32301
(904) 224-2469

Panhandle Medical Society
Cindy Mathis, Executive Director
P.O. Box 566
Chipley, FL 32428
(904) 638-1610 ex. 122

Parkinson's Support Group of Tallahassee
816 Piedmont Dr.
Tallahassee, FL 32312
(904) 385-0404

Senior Community Services Employment Program
1801 S. Gadsden St., #6
Tallahassee, FL 32301
(904) 224-0220

Senior Society Planning Council
2518 W. Tennessee St.
Tallahassee, FL 32304
(904) 575-9694

Senior Society Planning Council Adult Day Program
(Tallahassee) (904) 575-9694

Silver-Haired Legislature
1951 Meridian Rd., #84
Tallahassee, FL 32303
(904) 385-3865

Social Security Administration
227 N. Bronough St., #2070
Tallahassee, FL 32301
(904) 681-7139

Tallahassee Senior Citizens Center
1400 N. Monroe St.
Tallahassee, FL 32303
(904) 891-4000

Telephone Counseling and Referral Service
P.O. Box 20169
Tallahassee, FL 32316
(904) 224-6333

Veterans' Administration Outpatient Clinic
1607 St. James Ct.
Tallahassee, FL 32308
(904) 878-0191

Veterans' Affairs
(Tallahassee) (800) 827-1000

Veterans Service Office
Northwood Center
1940 N. Monroe St.
Tallahassee, FL 32303
(904) 488-8462

PSA III

Mid Florida Area Agency on Aging
Dean LaFrentz, Executive Director
5700 S.W. 34th Street, Ste. 222
Gainesville, FL 32608

Hamilton, Suwannee, Dixie, Lafayette, Columbia, Levy, Gilchrist, Union, Bradford, Alachua, Putnam, Citrus, Marion, Sumter, Hernando, Lake

American Association of Retired Persons (AARP)
Rt. 3, Box 493
Live Oak, FL 32060
(904) 362-5006

Alachua County Medical Society
Peggy J. Davenport, Executive Director
235 S.W. 2nd Ave.
Gainesville, FL 32601
(904)376-0715

Alzheimer's Association/North-Central Florida Chapter
502 N.W. 75th St., Suite 397
Gainesville, FL 32607
(904) 372-6266

Alzheimer's Association, Northeast Florida Chapter
2131 Mango Pl.
Jacksonville, FL 32207
(904) 398-5193

Alzheimer's Family Support Group (Hernando)
Seven Hills Plaza, 1244 Mariner Blvd.
Spring Hill, FL 34606
(904) 683-2994

Bradford County Medical Society
Maggie Phillips, Executive Secretary
P.O. Box 1060
Starke, FL 32091

Citrus County Medical Society
Trudy Elliott, Executive Secretary
P.O. Box 2601 (32751)
403 W. Highland Blvd.
Inverness, FL 32652-4756
(904) 344-3822

Columbia County Medical Society
601 Circle Dr., Suite 2-A
Lake City, FL 32055-4004
(904)758-3677

Commodities Program
P.O. Box 448
Bronson, FL 32621
(904) 486-4311

Commodities Program
Coliseum Complex
Live Oak, FL 32060
(904) 362-6079

Community Care for the Elderly
Advent Christian Village
Dowling Park, FL 32060
(904) 658-3333

Dixie County Medical Society
311 E. Ash St.
Perry, FL 32347

Disabled American Veterans
226 Parshley St.
Live Oak, FL 32060
(904) 362-1701

Extension Homemakers Office
1302 11th St., S.W.
Live Oak, FL 32060
(904) 362-2771

Food Stamp Office
Hwy. 27 N.
Mayo, FL 32066
(904) 294-1800

Food Stamp Office
501 S.E. Demorest St.
Live Oak, FL 32060
(904) 362-4429

Hamilton County Medical Society
Andrew Bass, President
315 S. Scriven Ave.
Lake Oak, FL 32060
(904) 362-4822

Hernando County Medical Society
Kate Lacey, Executive Director
12395 Cortez Blvd.
Brooksville, FL 34613
(904) 597-4690

Hernando-Pasco Hospice
12107 Majestic Blvd.
Hudson, FL 34667
(813) 863-7971

Hospice of Citrus County
3350 W. Audubon Park-Path
Lecanto, FL 33461-8450
(904) 527-2020

Hospice of Lake & Sumter
12300 Lane Park Rd.
Tavares, FL 32778
(904) 343-1341, ext. 201

Hospice of Marion County
P.O. Box 4860
Ocala, FL 34478
(904) 694-7158

Hospice of North Central Florida
801 S.W. 2nd Ave.
Gainesville, FL 32601
(904) 378-2121

HRS Aging and Adult Services
Jim Godwin, Program Administrator
1000 N.E. 16th Ave.
Bldg. 1, Rm. 144
Gainesville, FL 32601
(904) 336-5313

HRS Background Screening Coordinator
1000 N.E. 16th Ave., Bldg. J
Gainesville, FL 32609-4598

HRS District Administrator
1000 N.E. 16th Ave., Bldg. H
Gainesville, FL 32601
(904) 336-5010

HRS Human Services Program Specialist
(Medicaid eligibility determination)
Building A, Rm. 151
1000 N.E. 16th Ave.
Gainesville, FL 32609
(904) 336-5313

Lafayette County Medical Society
315 S. Scriven Ave.
Live Oak, FL 32060

Lake County Medical Society
Barbara Martin, Executive Director
P.O. Box 492740
Leesburg, FL 34749-2740

Long-Term Care Ombudsman Council
Donna Jackson, Coordinator
1000 N.E. 16th Ave., Bldg. H
Gainesville, FL 32609
(904) 336-5015, (800) 342-9004

Marion County Medical Society
Debbie R. Trammell, Executive Director
P.O. Box 3655
Ocala, FL 32678-3655

Mid-Florida Area Agency on Aging
Dean LaFrentz, Executive Director
5700 S.W. 34th St., Suite 222
Gainesville, FL 32608
(904) 378-6649

Physician's Referral Service
(904) 755-3503 (call collect)

Putnam County Medical Society
c/o Putnam Community Hospital
P.O. Drawer 778
Palatka, FL 32178

Senior Services
P.O. Box 70
Live Oak, FL 32060
(904) 294-2202

Sumter County Medical Society
Trudy Elliott, Executive Secretary
403 W. Highland Blvd.
Inverness, FL 32652-4756

Suwannee-Hamilton-Lafayette County Medical Society
315 S. Scriven Ave.
Live Oak, FL 32060

Three Rivers Legal Services, Inc.
817 W. Duval St.
Lake City, FL 32055
(904) 752-5960

Union County Medical Society
Peggy J. Davenport, Executive Director
235 S.W. 2nd Ave.
Gainesville, FL 32601

United Way Information and Referral
P.O. Box 938
Gainesville, Fl 32602-0938

Veterans Administration Medical Center
1601 S.W. Archer Rd.
Gainesville, FL 32606
(904) 376-1611

Veterans Administration Medical Center Support Group
801 S. Marion St.
Lake City, FL 32055
(904) 755-3016
Veterans Service Office
224 Pine Ave., Rm. 102
Live Oak, FL 32060
(904) 362-6869

Veteran's Administration Hospital
S. Marion St.
Lake City, FL 32055
(904) 755-3016

PSA IV

Northeast Florida Area Agency on Aging
Elizabeth Lee, Director
P.O. Box 43187
Jacksonville, FL 32203
(904) 388-6495

Baker, Nassau, Duval, Clay, St. Johns, Flagler, Volusia

Alzheimer's Association
310 N. Nova Rd.
Ormond Beach, FL 32174
(904) 673-8833

Alzheimer's Association/NE Florida Chapter
2131 Mango Pl.
Jacksonville, FL 32207
(904) 398-5193

Alzheimer's Care Management Program
2311 River Blvd.
Jacksonville, FL 32204
(904) 381-4839

Alzheimer's Resources Assistance and Education
The Extended Family
P.O. Box 10174
Daytona Beach, FL 32120
(904) 252-2489

Alzheimer's Support Group/NW Jacksonville
5626 Soutel Dr.
Jacksonville, FL 32219
(904) 765-0264

Baker County Senior Center
101 E. Macclenny Ave.
Macclenny, FL 32063
(904) 259-2223

Clay County Medical Society
P.O. Box 416
Orange Park, FL 32067
(904) 276-4966

Department of Insurance, Consumer Services
1104-H Beville Rd.
Daytona Beach, FL 32114
(904) 254-3920
or
111 Coastline Drive East
Suite 439, Box 40
Jacksonville, FL 32202
(904) 359-6146

Duval County Medical Society
Philip H. Gilbert, Executive Vice President
515 Lomax St.
Jacksonville, FL 32204

Flagler County Medical Society
P.O. Box 727
Bunnell, FL 32210
(904) 437-7300

Flagler County Senior Center
1000 Belle Terre Blvd.
Palm Coast, FL 32037
(904) 437-7300

Hospice of Northeast Florida
841 Prudential Dr.
Jacksonville, FL 32207
(904) 398-4724

Hospice of Volusia/Flagler
655 N. Clyde Morris Blvd.
Daytona Beach, FL 32114
(904) 257-6111

HRS Human Services Program Specialist
(Medicaid eligibility determinations)
5920 Arlington Expressway
P.O. Box 2417
Jacksonville, FL 32231-0083
(904) 723-5367

HRS Background Screening Coordinator
5920 Arlington Expressway
P.O. Box 2417
Jacksonville, FL 32231

HRS District Administrator
Lee Johnson
P.O. Box 2417-F
Jacksonville, FL 32231
(904) 723-2022

Keystone Senior Center
Commercial Circle
Keystone Heights, FL 32656
(904) 473-2065

Lane/Wiley Senior Center
6710 Wiley Rd.
Jacksonville, FL 32210
(904) 783-6589

Long-Term Care Ombudsman Council
Mark Thacker, Coordinator
5920 Arlington Expressway
P.O. Box 2417
Jacksonville, FL 32231
(904) 723-2058

Methodist Hospital Hospice
580 W. 8th St.
Jacksonville, FL 32209
(904) 798-8340

Nassau County Medical Society
205 1/2 Centre St.
Fernandina Beach, FL 32034
(904) 261-3407

New Smyrna Council on Aging
505 Canal St.
New Smyrna, FL 32168
(904) 427-3877

Senior Social Services Project
1133 Ionia St.
Jacksonville, FL 32206
(904) 630-0932

Mary L. Singleton Center
150 E. 1st St.
Jacksonville, FL 32206
(904) 630-0995

St. Johns County Medical Society
P.O. Box 100
400 Health Park Blvd.
St. Augustine, FL 32086

St. Johns Senior Center
11 Old Mission Ave.
St. Augustine, FL 32084
(904) 824-1648

Veterans Administration Hospital
1900 Mason Ave.
Daytona Beach, FL 32117-5115
(904) 274-4600

Volusia County Medical Society
Gloria S. Barkin, Executive Director
303 N. Clyde Morris Blvd.
P.O. Box 9595
Daytona Beach, FL 32120

Westside Senior Center
1083 Line St.
Jacksonville, FL 32210
(904) 630-0724

Woodland Acres Senior Center
8200 Kona Ave.
Jacksonville, FL 32211
(904) 725-0624

PSA V

Area Agency on Aging
Sally Gronda, Director
Tampa Bay Regional Planning Council
9455 Koger Blvd.,
   Hendry Bldg.
St. Petersburg, FL 33702
(813) 577-5151

Pasco, Pinellas

AARP Prescription Service
6500 N. 34th St.
St. Petersburg, FL 33733
(800) 522-0531

Alzheimer's Disease Support Group, CARES
7505 Rottingham Rd.
Port Richey, FL 34668-2648
(813) 862-9291

Alzheimer's/Parkinson Support Group of Dade City
Humana Hospital-Pasco
Dade City, FL 33525
(904) 521-3034

Bethlehem Center at St. Jerome's Church Support Group
10895 Hamlin Blvd.
Largo, FL 34644
(813) 595-4610

Central Gulfside Hospice
6230 Lafayette St.
New Port Richey, FL 34652
(813) 845-5707

Department of Insurance, Consumer Services
3160 5th Ave. N., Suite 135
St. Petersburg, FL 33713
(813) 893-2351

Directions for Mental Health
1437 S. Belcher Rd., Suite 200
Clearwater, FL 34624
(813) 536-5950

Hernando-Pasco Hospice
12107 Majestic Blvd.
Hudson, FL 34667
(813) 863-7971

HRS Aging and Adult Services
Pat Bell, Program Administrator
11351 Ulmerton Rd
Largo, FL 34648-1630
(813) 588-6600

HRS Background Screening Coordinator
11351 Ulmerton Rd., Suite 100
Largo, FL 34648-1630
(813) 588-6600

HRS District Administrator
11351 Ulmerton Rd., Suite 100
Largo, FL 34648-1630
(813) 588-6600

HRS Human Services Program Specialist
(Medicaid eligibility determinations)
11351 Ulmerton Rd., Suite 100
Largo, FL 34648-1630
(813) 588-6600

HRS Human Services Program Specialist
(Medicaid eligibility determinations)
701 94th Avenue North
St. Petersburg, FL 33702
(813) 588-6915

Lealman Day Care Center Support Group
3455 58th Ave. N.
St. Petersburg, FL 33714
(813) 527-5212

Long-Term Care Ombudsman Council
Ann White, Coordinator
701 94th Ave. N.
St. Petersburg, FL 33702
(813) 576-0035

Pasco County Medical Society
Joy P. Imperato, Executive Director
10934 U.S. Hwy. 19, Suite 205
Port Richey, FL 34668-2565

Pinellas County Medical Society
William E. Coletti, Executive Director
7411 114th Ave. N., Suite 306
Largo, FL 34643

Significant Others Support Groups
210 Ewing Ave.
Clearwater, FL 34616
(813) 443-1560

Suncoast Center for Community Mental Health Support Group
4024 Central Ave.
St. Petersburg, FL 33711
(813) 327-7656

Veterans' Affairs
(St. Petersburg/Clearwater) (813) 898-2121

PSA VI

West Central Florida Area Agency on Aging
Maureen Sherman-Kelly, Director
1419 W. Waters Ave., Suite 114
Tampa, FL 33604
(813) 933-5945

Hillsborough, Manatee, Polk, Highlands, Hardee

Adult Children of Aging Parents/FMHI Support Group
13301 N. Bruce B. Downs Blvd.
Tampa, FL 33612
(813) 974-4665

Alzheimer's Association/Greater Tampa Chapter
2700 N. MacDill Ave., #205
Tampa, FL 33607-2273
(813) 875-7766

American Association of Retired Persons (AARP)
Chapter Information (813) 576-1155
Membership Information (800) 441-2277

Department of Insurance, Consumer Services
1313 N. Tampa St., Suite 809
Tampa, FL 33602
(813) 272-2330

Florida Mental Health Institute (FMHI)
13301 N. Bruce B. Downs Blvd.
Tampa, FL 33612
(813) 974-4665

Good Shepherd Hospice of Mid-Florida
P.O. Box 7129
Winter Haven, FL 33883
(813) 297-1880

Hardee County Medical Society
Jeani Ferguson, Executive Secretary
c/o Florida Power & Light
14 E. Oak St., P.O. Box 431
Arcadia, FL 33821
(813) 494-1511

Hillsborough County Medical Society
Thomas B. Clark, Executive Vice President
606 S. Blvd.
Tampa, FL 33606

Highlands County Medical Society
Lori B. Olson, Executive Secretary
11 W. Thomas St., P.O. Box 310
Avon Park, FL 33825

Hospice of Hillsborough
3010 Azeele St.
Tampa, FL 33609
(813) 877-2200

HRS Human Services Program Specialist
(Medicaid eligibility determinations)
4000 W. Dr. Martin Luther King Jr. Blvd.
Tampa, FL 33614
(813) 871-7660

HRS Aging and Adult Services
Dorothy Dexter, Program Administrator
4000 W. Dr. Martin Luther King Jr. Blvd.
Tampa, FL 33614
(813) 871-7660

HRS Background Screening Coordinator
4000 W. Dr. Martin Luther King Jr. Blvd.
Tampa, FL 33614

HRS District Administrator
4000 W. Dr. Martin Luther King Jr. Blvd.
Tampa, FL 33614
(813) 871-7444

Lakeland Multi-Purpose Senior Center Support Group
1200 Southern Ave.
Lakeland, FL 33801
(813) 499-2606

Long-Term Care Ombudsman Council
Marion Chadwick, Coordinator
8900 N. Armenia St., Bldg. 200, Suite I
Tampa, FL 33604
(813) 935-7084

Manatee County Medical Society
Mary J. Beihl, Executive Director
2722 Manatee Ave., W.
Bradenton, FL 34205

Polk County Medical Association
Elsie M. Trask, Executive Director
402 S. Kentucky Ave., Suite 350
P.O. Box 927
Lakeland, FL 33802

St. Joseph's Hospital Alzheimer's Support Group
3001 W. Martin Luther King Jr. Blvd.
Tampa, FL 33677
(813) 870-4440

Suncoast Alzheimer's Information Line
USF Health Sciences Center
12901 N. Bruce B. Downs Blvd., MDC 50
Tampa, FL 33612
(800) 633-4563

Suncoast Gerontology Center, Memory Disorder Clinic
USF Health Sciences Center
12901 N. Bruce B. Downs Blvd. MDC 50
Tampa, FL 33612
(813) 974-4355

Temple Terrace Presbyterian Church Stroke Support Group
420 Bullard Pkwy.
Temple Terrace, FL 33617
(813) 988-3514

Veterans' Affairs
(Tampa) (813) 299-0451

PSA VII

Area Agency on Aging
Judy Thames, Director
East Central Florida Regional Planning Council
1011 Wymore Rd., Suite 207
Winter Park, FL 32789-1330
(407) 623-1075

Seminole, Orange, Osceola, Brevard

Alzheimer's Resource Center Information Line
250 Loch Lomond
P.O. Box 1153
Winter Park, FL 32792
(800) 330-1910

Alzheimer's Association, Inc./Orlando Chapter
(407) 422-9595

Alzheimer's Association Support Groups
1250 S. Harbor City Blvd., #31
Melbourne, FL 32901
(407) 729-8536

Alzheimer's Resource Center Information Line
250 Loch Lomond
P.O. Box 1153
Winter Park, FL 32792
(800) 330-1910

Directory

Senior Center Alzheimer's Support Group
1099 Shady Ln.
Kissimmee, FL 32743
(407) 847-4357

Brevard County Community Services Council *(Transportation)*
1149 Lake Dr.
Cocoa, FL 32922
(407) 631-2744

Brevard County Medical Society
Christine Welch, Executive Director
110 Barton Ave.
Rockledge, FL 32955

Brevard Hospice
110 Longwood Ave.
P.O. Box 560965
Rockledge, FL 32956
(407) 636-2211, ext. 2720

Central Brevard Support Group
1175 Buddy Ct.
Rockledge, FL 32955
(407) 636-7286

Crisis Center
300 S. Bay Ave.
Sanford, FL 32771
(407) 321-4357

Community Service Council-Senior Activity Program
1149 Lake Dr.
Cocoa, FL 32922
(407) 631-2744

Creative Care Center
3300 N. Atlantic Ave.
Cocoa Beach, FL 32931
(407) 784-3502

Crises Services of Brevard *(24 hours)*
P.O. Box 56-1108
Rockledge, FL 32956-1108
(407) 631-8944

Department of Insurance, Consumer Services
400 W. Robinson St., Suite 401
Orlando, FL 32801
(407) 423-6105

Better Living For Seniors
636 Florida Central Pkwy.
Longwood, FL 32750
(407) 831-1631, (407) 831-4357

Florida Living Nursing Center
3355 E. Semoran Blvd.
Apopka, FL 32703
(407) 862-6263

Hispanic Support Group/Englewood Neighborhood Center
6123 La Costa Dr.
Orlando, FL 32807
(407) 843-1910

Holmes Regional Hospice
1900 Bairy Rd.
West Melborne, FL 32904
(407) 952-0494

Hospice of Central Florida
2500 Maitland Ctr. Pkwy., Suite 300
Orlando, FL 32751
(407) 875-0028

Hospice of Central Florida-Osceola
2200 Irlo Bronson Memorial Hwy.
Kissimmee, FL 32741
(407) 846-7444

Hospice of the Treasure Coast
P.O. Box 1742
602 Atlantic Ave.
Fort Pierce, FL 34954
(407) 465-0504

HRS Aging and Adult Services
Robert Bridger, Program Administrator
400 W. Robinson St., Suite 912
Orlando, FL 32801
(407) 423-6240

HRS Background Screening Coordinator
509 South Park Ave.
Apopka, FL 32703

HRS District Administrator
400 W. Robinson St., Suite 809
Orlando, FL 32801
(407) 423-6208

HRS Human Services Program Specialist
(Medicaid eligibility determinations)
400 W. Robinson St., Suite 912
Orlando, FL 32801
(407) 423-6240

Human Services Council Information and Referral Center
3191 Maguire, #150
Orlando, FL 32803
(407) 897-6464

Loch Lomond Support Group
250 Loch Lommond
P.O. Box 1153
Winter Park, FL 32790-1153
(407) 678-3334

Memory Disorder Clinic
Florida Institute of Technology
Claude Pepper Institute for Aging and Therapeutic Research
1322 S. Oak St.
Melbourne, FL 32901-3111
(407) 768-9575

Long-Term Care Ombudsman Council
Nancy Kesecker, Coordinator
400 W. Robinson St., Suite 912
Orlando, FL 32801
(407) 423-6114

North Brevard Hospice
9 S. Palm Ave.
Titusville, FL 32796
(407) 269-4240

Osceola County Council on Aging
1099 Shady Ln.
Kissimmee, FL 32743
(407) 846-8532

Orange County Medical Society
Ron L. Fitzwater, Executive Vice President
1851 W. Colonial Dr., Suite 200
Orlando, FL 32804

Osceola County Family Support Group
1099 Shady Ln.
Kissimmee, FL 32743
(407) 846-8532

Osceola County Medical Society
Lee Lamb, Executive Secretary
P.O. Box 421613
Kissimmee, FL 34742-1613

Palm Bay Methodist Church Support Group
2100 Port Malabar Blvd. N.E.
Palm Bay, FL 32905
(407) 727-8651

Park Care Senior Day Center
230 North Perth Ln.
Winter Park, FL 32792
(407) 629-5771

Sanford Alzheimer Family Support Group
200 W. Airport Blvd.
Sanford, FL 32771
(407) 843-1910, (800) 330-1910

Seminole Community Day Treatment
2462 Park Ave.
Sanford, FL 32771
(407) 323-2036

Seminole County Medical Society
Rona Snyder, Executive Secretary
P.O. Box 2283
Sanford, FL 32772

St. Mary Magdalene Catholic Church
710 Spring Lake Rd.
Altamonte Springs, FL 32701
(407) 831-9630

Titusville Nursing/Convalescent Center Support Group
1705 Jess Parrish Ct.
Titusville, FL 32796
(407) 269-5720

United Methodist Church Support Group
450 Lee Ave., #5
Satellite Beach, FL 32901
(407) 777-0116

United Methodist Church Support Group
1935 S. Fiske Blvd.
Rockledge, FL 32955
(407) 632-7387

Directory

Veterans' Affairs
(Cocoa/Cocoa Beach) (407) 633-2012
(Melbourne) (407) 633-2199
(Orlando) (407) 425-7521

Veteran's Service Office
Melbourne (407) 242-6512
Merritt Island (407) 633-2012
Titusville (407) 264-5219
Osceola County (407) 847-1288
Seminole County (407) 323-4330

Visiting Nurse Association/Community Care for Elderly Program
1655 Peel Ave.
Orlando, FL 32806
(407) 894-4669

Wesley United Methodist Church Support Group
2075 Minton Rd.
Melbourne, FL 32901
(407) 727-7585

West Orange Manor Support Group
411 N. Dillard St.
Winter Garden, FL 34787
(407) 656-3810

Widowed Persons Service
(407) 649-9209

Winter Park Family Support Group
Stratford Square Apts.
Howell Branch Rd.
Winter Park, FL 32792
(407) 843-1910

PSA VIII

South Central Florida Area Agency on Aging
Dr. Wallace Hunter, Director
140 Jackson St.
Fort Myers, FL 33901
(813) 332-4233

DeSoto, Charlotte, Lee, Glades, Hendry, Sarasota, Collier

Alzheimer's Association
350 Braden Ave.
Bradenton, FL 34243
(813) 355-7637

Alzheimer's Association
2789 Ortiz S.E.
Ft. Myers, FL 33905
(813) 355-7637

Alzheimer's Association
666 Tamiami Tr. N. #37
Naples, FL 33940
(813) 624-5722

Alzheimer's Association
118 Sullivan St.
Punta Gorda, FL 33950
(813) 634-5727

Charlotte County Medical Society
Regina Manganiello, Executive Secretary
C & S Bank Bldg.
3195 Tamiami Tr.
Port Charlotte, FL 33952

Collier County Medical Society
Christine J. Kyle, Executive Secretary
P.O. Box 2102
Naples, FL 33939

Department of Insurance, Consumer Services
2295 Victoria Ave., Suite 163
Fort Myers, FL 33901
(813) 332-6948

DeSoto-Hardee-Glades County Medical Society
Jeani Ferguson, Executive Secretary
c/o Florida Power & Light
14 E. Oak St., P.O. Box 431
Arcadia, FL 33821

Glades County Medical Society
Jeani Ferguson, Executive Secretary
c/o Florida Power & Light
14 E. Oak St., P.O. Box 431
Arcadia, FL 33821

Hendry County Medical Society
Jean Wicken, Executive Director
3540 Forest Hill Blvd., Suite 101
West Palm Beach, FL 33406

Hope Hospice
8290 College Pkwy., Suite 100
Fort Myers, FL 33919
(813) 482-4673

Hospice of Naples
1095 Whippoorwill Ln.
Naples, FL 33999
(813) 261-4404

Hospice of Southwest Florida
6055 Rand Blvd.
Sarasota, FL 34238
(813) 923-5822

HRS Aging and Adult Services
Carol Hall, Program Administrator
P.O. Box 60085
Fort Myers, FL 33906
(813) 338-1392

HRS Background Screening Coordinator
6719 Winkler Rd.
P.O. Box 60085
Fort Myers, FL 33906

HRS District Administrator
P.O. Box 60085
Fort Myers, FL 33906
(813) 338-1392

HRS Human Services Program Specialist
(Medicaid eligibility determinations)
2295 Victoria Ave.
P.O. Box 60085
Fort Myers, FL 33901
(813) 338-1392

Lee County Medical Society
Ann Wilks, Executive Director
3806 Fowler St., Suite 2 (33901)
P.O. Box 06041
Fort Myers, FL 33906-6041

Lee Memorial Hospital/Alzheimer's Support Group, Older Adult Services
2776 Cleveland Ave.
P.O. Drawer 2218
Fort Myers, FL 33902
(813) 332-1111

Long-Term Care Ombudsman Council
Anne Gordon, Coordinator
P.O. Box 60085
Fort Myers, FL 33906
(813) 433-6702/6703

Pinebrook Place Healthcare Center
1240 Pinebrook Rd.
Venice, FL 34292
(813) 371-5895

Alzheimer Hotline
(800) 621-0379

Sarasota County Medical Society
Beckett J. Shady-King, Executive Director
23 Webb St.
Osprey, FL 34229

Sarasota Memorial/Caregivers Support, Training Program
1200 S. Tamiami Tr.
Sarasota, FL 34239
(813) 957-7416

Suncoast Alzheimer's Information Line (SAIL) *(Crystal River to Naples)*
(800) 663-4563

Veterans' Affairs
(Fort Myers) (800) 827-2204
(Sarasota) (813) 951-5498

Directory

PSA IX

Area Agency on Aging of Palm Beach/Treasure Coast, Inc.
Laura Landwirth, Executive Director
8895 N. Military Tr., Suite 201-C
Palm Beach Gardens, FL 33410
(407) 694-7601

Indian River, Okeechobee, St. Lucie, Martin, Palm Beach

Adult Day Care, North County Alzheimer's Support Group
5217 W. Lake Park Rd.
West Palm Beach, FL 33410
(407) 627-6488

Alzheimer's Disease and Related Disorders Association
3200 N. Federal Hwy., #226
Boca Raton, FL 33431
(407) 392-1363, (407) 736-2699

Alzheimer's/Parkinson's Disease Support Group
P.O. Box 1465
Vero Beach, FL 32961
(407) 563-0505

Bethesda Memorial Hospital Support Group
2815 S. Seacrest Blvd.
Boynton Beach, FL 33435
(407) 737-7733

Deaf Service Center of Palm Beach County, Inc.
5730 Corporate Way, #230
West Palm Beach, FL 33407
(407) 478-3903
TDD (407) 478-3904

Department of Insurance, Consumer Services
111 Georgia Ave., Suite 209
West Palm Beach, FL 33401
(407) 837-5045

Division of Blind Services
111 Georgia Ave., Rm. 101
West Palm Beach, FL 33401
(407) 837-5026

Division of Senior Services
810 Datura St., #301, C-2
West Palm Beach, FL 33401
(407) 355-4782

Hispanic Human Resources Council
1427 S. Congress Ave.
West Palm Beach, FL 33406
(407) 641-7400

Hospice by the Sea
1531 W. Palmetto Park Rd.
Boca Raton, FL 33486
(407) 395-5031

Hospice of Martin
2300 S.E. Ocean Blvd.
Stuart, FL 34996
(407) 287-7860

Hospice of Okeechobee
P.O. Box 1548
Okeechobee, FL 34972
(813) 467-2321

Hospice of Palm Beach County
5300 East Ave.
West Palm Beach, FL 33407
(407) 848-5200, ext. 211

HRS Aging and Adult Services
Lois Peterson, Program Administrator
111 Georgia Ave.
West Palm Beach, FL 33401
(407) 837-5138

HRS Background Screening Coordinator
111 Georgia Ave.
West Palm Beach, FL 33401

HRS District Administrator
111 Georgia Ave.
West Palm Beach, FL 33401
(407) 837-5138

HRS Human Services Program Specialist
(Medicaid eligibility determinations)
2701 Lake Ave.
West Palm Beach, FL 33405
(407) 837-5340

Indian River Council on Aging
P.O. Box 2102, 694, 14th St.
Vero Beach, FL 32961-2102
(407) 569-0760

Indian River County Medical Society
Ann Thomas, Executive Director
2300 Third Ct., Suite F
P.O. Box 573
Vero Beach, FL 32961

Jewish Community Center
3151 N. Military Tr.
West Palm Beach, FL 33409
(407) 689-7700, (407) 395-8920

Jewish Family and Children's Service Support Group
4605 Commerce Dr.
West Palm Beach, FL 33417
(407) 684-1991

Jupiter Hospital Support Group
1220 S. Old Dixie Hwy.
Jupiter, FL 33458
(407) 747-2234

North County Day Care
5217 W. Lake Park Rd.
West Palm Beach, FL 33410
(407) 627-6488

Legal Aid Society of Palm Beach County
224 Datura St., #301
West Palm Beach, FL 33401
(407) 655-8944

Liberty Inn Alzheimer's Support Group
5858 Heritage Park Way
Delray Beach, FL 33484
(407) 499-2500

Long-Term Care Ombudsman Council
Claudette Connors, Coordinator
111 Georgia Ave.
West Palm Beach, FL 33401
(407) 837-5038

Mae Volen Senior Center
1515 W. Palmetto Park Rd.
P.O. Box 2468
Boca Raton, FL 33427-2468
(407) 736-3820

Martin Council on Aging
P.O. Box 3029
Stuart, FL 34995
(407) 283-8026

Martin County Medical Society
Pat Kelly, Executive Secretary
c/o Martin Memorial Hospital
P.O. Box 9010
Stuart, FL 34995

Martin Memorial Hospital Alzheimer's Support Group
P.O. Box 9010
Stuart, FL 34996
(407) 288-5848

Meadowbrook Residential Care Center Support Group
1130 N.W. 15th St.
Boca Raton, FL 33432
(407) 392-1363

Mental Health Association
909 Fern St.
West Palm Beach, FL 33409
(407) 832-3755

Mid-County Day Care
202 N. "H" St.
Lake Worth, FL 33460
(407) 586-6123

Mid-County Senior Center
202 N. "H" St.
Lakes Wales, FL 33460
(407) 586-6102

Noreen-McKeen Residence for Geriatric Care Support Group
315 S. Flagler Dr.
West Palm Beach, FL 33401
(407) 655-8544

North County Senior Citizen Center Support Group
5217 N. Lake Blvd.
West Palm Beach, FL 33418
(407) 627-6470

North County Senior Citizen Center
5217 N. Lake Park Rd.
West Palm Beach, FL 33418
(407) 736-2699

Northeast Alzheimer Day Care Center
227 N.W. 2nd St.
Deerfield Beach, FL 33441
(305) 480-4460

Okeechobee Council on Aging
1019 W. South Park St.
Okeechobee, FL 34972-4758
(813) 763-7644

Okeechobee County Medical Society
Shirley E. Morgan, Executive Secretary
P.O. Box 3719
Fort Pierce, FL 34948

Palm Beach County Division of Senior Services
202 N. "H" St.
Lake Worth, FL 33461
(407) 586-6123

Palm Beach County Medical Society
Jean Wicken, Executive Director
3540 Forest Hill Blvd., Suite 101
West Palm Beach, FL 33406

Respite Catholic Charities
9995 N. Military Tr.
Palm Beach Gardens, FL 33410
(407)775-9576

Ruth Rales Jewish Family Service
902 Clint Moore Rd., #208
Boca Raton, FL 33487
(407) 994-5678

Senior Aides/Employment
810 Datura St.
West Palm Beach, FL 33402
(407) 355-4782

Senior District Office
5217 N. Lake Blvd.
Palm Beach Gardens, FL
(407) 627-5765
 and
202 N. "11" St.
Lake Worth, FL
(407) 586-6155

Senior Services(*Transportation*)
West Palm Beach
(407) 820-4734

St. Andrews Medical Center Support Group
6152 N. Verde Tr.
Boca Raton, FL 33433
(407) 487-5200

St. Lucie Council on Aging
1505 Orange Ave.
Fort Pierce, FL 34950-6899
(407) 465-5220

St. Lucie-Okeechobee County Medical Society
Shirley E. Morgan, Executive Secretary
P.O. Box 3719
Fort Pierce, FL 34948

Treasure Coast Senior Services
601 Boston Ave.
Fort Pierce, FL 34950
(407) 465-3108

VNA Hospice of Indian River County
1111 36th St.
Vero Beach, FL 32960
(407) 567-5551

West Boca United Methodist Church Support Group
9087 W. Glades Rd.
Boca Raton, FL 33428
(407) 482-7335

PSA X

Area Agency on Aging of Broward County
Edith Lederberg, Executive Director
5345 N.W. 35th Ave.
Fort Lauderdale, FL 33309
(305) 485-6370

Broward

Alzheimer's Association (Broward Chapter)
8333 W. McNab Rd., #203
Tamarac, FL 33321
(305) 726-0002

Alzheimer Day Care
6009 N.W. 10th St.
Margate, FL 33063
(305) 977-6556
(305) 981-2283, (weekend)

Alzheimer's Family Center, Inc.
4900 W. Atlantic Blvd, #4
Margate, FL 33063
(305) 971-7155

Alzheimer's In-Home Respite (Southeast)
3081 Taft St.
Hollywood, FL 33021
(305) 987-3987

Arthritis Foundation
915 Little River Dr., Suite 401
Fort Lauderdale, FL 33304
(305) 563-0027

Beta Senior Employment Program
330 N. Andrews Ave.
Fort Lauderdale, FL 33301
(305) 765-4541

Broward Alzheimer's Coordinating Council/Area Agency on Aging
5345 N.W. 35th Ave.
Fort Lauderdale, FL 33309
(305) 485-6370

Broward Center for the Blind
650 N. Andrews Ave.
Fort Lauderdale, FL 33311
(305) 463-4217

Broward County Council of Senior Citizens
7787 Gulf Circle Dr.
Margate, FL 33063
(305) 971-9681

Broward County Elderly Services
115 S. Andrews Ave., Rm. 516
Fort Lauderdale, FL 33301
(305) 357-6765

Broward County Elderly Services
311 A, N.E. 3rd St.
Fort Lauderdale, FL 33301
(305) 522-2556

Broward County Medical Association
Cynthia Peterson, Executive Vice President
5101 N.W. 21st Ave., Suite 510
P.O. Box 8457
Fort Lauderdale, FL 33310

Catholic Community Services
1300 S. Andrews Ave.
Fort Lauderdale, FL 33336
(305) 522-2513

Department of Insurance, Consumer Services
200 S.E. 6th St., Suite 404
Fort Lauderdale, FL 33301
(305) 467-4339

Family Services Agency, Inc.
3830 S.W. 2nd Ct.
Fort Lauderdale, FL 33312
(305) 587-7880

First Call for Help Line
P.O. Box 14428
Fort Lauderdale, FL 33302
(305) 522-5220

Florida Division of Blind Services
3075 W. Oakland Park Blvd., #211
Fort Lauderdale, FL 33311
(305) 497-3360

Foster Grandparent Program
5975 W. Sunrise Blvd., # 208 B
Fort Lauderdale, FL 33313
(305) 792-8589

Handicapped of South Broward, Inc.
117 Lone Pine Tr.
Pembroke Park, FL 33009
(305) 961-8286

Henderson Mental Health Center
 Gerontology Dept.
330 S.W. 27th Ave.
Fort Lauderdale, FL 33312
(305) 791-4300

Home Improvement
115 S. Andrews Ave., 335 U
Fort Lauderdale, FL 33301
(305) 357-6700

Home Touch Program
771 N.W. 22nd Rd.
Fort Lauderdale, FL 33311
(305) 792-1180

Hospice Care of Broward County
309 S.E. 18th St.
Fort Lauderdale, FL 33316
(305) 467-7423, ext. 22

Hospice of Gold Coast Home Health Services
911 E. Atlantic Blvd., Suite 200
Pompano Beach, FL 33060
(305) 785-2990, ext. 63

Hospice of Gold Coast
911 E. Atlantic Blvd., Suite 200
Pompano Beach, FL 33060
(305) 785-2990

Hospice Care of Broward County, Inc.
3323 W. Commercial Blvd., #200
Fort Lauderdale, FL 33309
(305) 486-4085

Housing Rehabilitation Program
2500 Hollywood Blvd., #314
Hollywood, FL 33020
(305) 921-3381

HRS Aging and Adult Services
Amemilo Maicas, Program Administrator
201 W. Broward Blvd.
Fort Lauderdale, FL 33301
(305) 467-4258

HRS Background Screening Coordinator
201 W. Broward Blvd., Rm. 306
Fort Lauderdale, FL 33301

HRS District Administrator
201 W. Broward Blvd.
Fort Lauderdale, FL 33301
(305) 467-4258

HRS Food Stamp Hotline
(800) 342-9274

HRS Food Stamp Central County
311 N. State Rd. 7
Plantation, FL 33317
(305) 797-8200

HRS Food Stamp North County
1801 W. Sample Rd.
Pompano Beach, FL 33064
(305) 969-3400

HRS Food Stamp South County
7261 Sheriden Street
West Hollywood, FL 33024
(305) 985-2780

HRS Human Services Program Specialist
(Medicaid eligibility determinations)
3800 Inverrary Blvd. Ste. 408
Fort Lauderdale, FL 33301
(305) 497-3353

Human Services Network, Inc.
4110 N. State Rd. 7
Fort Lauderdale, FL 33309
(305) 731-8770

Jewish Family Services of Broward County
3500 N. State Rd. 7
Fort Lauderdale, FL 33319
(305) 966-0956
 and
6100 Hollywood Blvd., #410
Fort Lauderdale, FL 33354
(305) 749-1505

Jewish Family Services of Broward-Respite Care
8358 W. Oakland Park Blvd.
Fort Lauderdale, FL 33351
(305) 749-7777

Legal Aid Service of Broward County
609 S.W. 1st Ave.
Fort Lauderdale, FL 33301
(305) 765-8955
and
1301 W. Copans Rd., Bldg A, Suite 2-N
Pompano Beach, FL 33064
(305) 975-7383

Library for the Blind and Visually Handicapped
100 S. Andrews Ave.
Fort Lauderdale, FL 33301
(305) 357-7555

L & M Placement Service
Statewide ACLF registry
5747 Park Rd., #202
Ft. Lauderdale, FL 33312
(800) 445-6565

Long-Term Care Ombudsman Council
Sandra Pavelka, Coordinator
1403 N.W. 40th Ave., Suite A
Lauderhill, FL 33313
(305) 467-4223

Miramar Satellite Senior Center
7667 Venetian St.
Miramar, FL 33023
(305) 973-0300

Match-Up Program
Northwest Focal Point Senior Center
5750 Park Dr.
Margate, FL 33063
(305) 973-4831

Medicaid Transportation
Sunrise Blvd. (north to Palm Beach County line)
(305) 797-8240
Sunrise Blvd. (south to Dade County line)
(305) 985-2780

Shopping Assistance Program
3201 West Copans Rd.
Pompano, FL 33069
(305) 357-6794

Social Service Transportation
(Wheelchair service)
57-C, N. Federal Hwy.
Fort Lauderdale, FL 33311
(305) 527-8645

Wheelchair Wagon
(Wheelchair service)
P.O. Box 2281
Hollywood, FL 33026
(305) 966-6548

Memory Disorder Center of South Florida
North Broward Medical Center
201 E. Sample Rd.
Pompano, FL 33064
(305) 786-7392

Mental Health Association of Broward and Center for Gerontology
5546 W. Oakland Blvd.
Lauderhill, FL 33313
(305) 733-3994

Miramar Satellite-Senior Center
7667 Venetian St.
Miramar, FL 33023
(305) 989-6200

Northeast Focal Point Senior Center
227 N.W. 2nd St.
Deerfield Beach, FL 33441
(305) 480-4449

Northwest Focal Point Senior Center
5750 Park Dr.
Margate, FL 33063
(305) 977-6556

North Broward Medical Center Memory Disorder Center of South Florida
201 Sample Rd.
Pompano, FL 33064
(305) 786-7392
(305) 786-2493 (support group)

Praxis Alzheimer's Care Campus
1431 S.W. 9th Ave.
Deerfield Beach, FL 33441
(305) 428-8544

Psychological Clinic-Nova University
311 University Dr., #307
Coral Springs, FL 33065
(305) 753-7020

Retired Senior Volunteer Program (RSVP)
1164 E. Oakland Park Blvd., #214
Fort Lauderdale, FL 33334
(305) 563-8991

The Samaritan Center
730 N.E. 4th Ave.
Fort Lauderdale, FL 33304
(305) 463-2273

Senior Aides Program
1164 E. Oakland Park Blvd.
Fort Lauderdale, FL 33334
(305) 563-8991

Senior Citizen Law Project
609 S.W. 1st Ave.
Fort Lauderdale, FL 33301
(305) 563-8558

Senior Community Service Employment
1100 E. Oakland Park Blvd.
Fort Lauderdale, FL 33334
(305) 561-9504

Southeast Focal Point-Meyerhoff Senior Center
3081 Taft St.
Hollywood, FL 33021
(305) 997-3987

Southeast Florida Center on Aging
Florida International University
North Miami Campus
North Miami, FL 33181
(305) 940-5550

Southeast Focal Point Alzheimer In-Home Respite Program
3081 Taft St.
Hollywood, FL 33021
(305) 987-3987

Southwest Focal Point Senior Center
6700 S.W. 13th St.
Pembroke Pines, FL 33023
(305) 981-2283

U.S. Railroad Retirement Board
299 E. Broward Blvd., #407
Fort Lauderdale, FL 33301
(305) 527-7372

United Hearing and Deaf Services, Inc.
4850 W. Oakland Park Blvd., #207
Fort Lauderdale, FL 33313
(305) 731-7200

University Community Hospital Alzheimer Support Group
7201 N. University Dr.
Tamarac, FL 33321
(305) 721-2200

Veterans' Affairs
(Fort Lauderdale/Hollywood)
(305) 522-4725

Veterans' Assistance Center
101 S.W. 1st Ave.
Fort Lauderdale, FL 33301
(305) 357-7560

Veterans Services Division
3550 Hollywood Blvd.
Hollywood, FL 33021
(305) 831-0420
   and
1600 W. Hillsborough
Deerfield Beach, FL 33442
(305) 831-1243

Widowed Persons Service
3000 N. University Dr.
Fort Lauderdale, FL 33316
(305) 733-3994

PSA XI

Alliance for Aging, Inc.
John Stokesberry, Executive Director
9100 S. Dadeland Blvd., Suite 400
Miami, FL 33156
(305) 670-6500

Dade, Monroe

ACTION
Transportation (City of Miami residents only)
(305) 545-9298

Advocate Seniors County Court Services
(305) 324-0550

Alzheimer's Association
Greater Miami Chapter
Kane Concourse
Bay Harbor Island, FL 33154
(305) 864-5866

Alzheimer's Careline at Miami Jewish Home & Hospital
5200 N.E. 2nd Ave.
Miami, FL 33137
(305) 576-5533, and toll free, nationwide (800) 726-6677

Alzheimer's Clinical Research Group
Baumel-Eisner Neuromedical Institute
1135 Kane Course, 3rd Floor
Bay Harbor Island, FL 33154
(305) 865-0063

Camillus House
726 N.E. 1st Ave.
Miami, FL 33132
(305) 374-1065

Center for Survival and Independent Living
1335 N.W. 14th St.
Miami, FL 33125
(305) 547-5444

Community Care Adult Day Care Center
151 N.E. 52nd St.
Miami, FL 33137
(305) 754-1996

County Elderly Services Division
111 N.W. 1st Ave., Suite 2210
Miami, FL 33128-1912
(305) 375-5335

Dade County Medical Association
Patricia Handler, Executive Vice President
1501 N.W. North River Dr.
Miami, FL 33125

Department of Insurance, Consumer Services
401 N.W. 2nd Ave., Suite N-307
Miami, FL 33128-1700
(305) 377-5235

Dial-A-Ride (Opa Locka only)
(305) 688-4611

Douglas Gardens-City Senior Adult Day Health Care Center
6447 N.E. 7th Ave.
Miami, FL 33138
(305) 754-1777

Downtown Senior Citizens Community Center
Gesu Church
118 N.E. 2nd Ave.
Miami, FL 33132
(305) 374-6099

Edison-Little River Adult Day Care Center
150 N.E. 79th St.
Miami, FL 33150
(305) 751-4342

Douglas Gardens/City of Miami Senior Adult Day Health Center
Legion Park
6447 N.E. 7th Ave.
Miami, FL 33138
(305) 754-1777

Douglas Gardens Ambulatory Health Center
151 N.E. 52nd St.
Miami, FL 33137
(305) 751-8626, Ext. 161

Douglas Gardens Community Mental Health Center
701 Lincoln Road Mall
Miami Beach, FL 33139
(305) 531-5341

The Leo Gelvan and Family Community Care Adult Day Health Center
5200 N.E. 2nd Ave.
Miami, FL 33137
(305) 754-1996

Geriatric Residential and Treatment Systems (GRTS)
1733 N.E. 162nd St.
North Miami Beach, FL 33162
(305) 945-5340

Goodlet Adult Center
(Hialeah)(305) 825-4947

Greater Miami Jewish Federation Information and Referral
4200 Biscayne Blvd.
Miami, FL 33137
(305) 576-4000

Gumenick Alzheimer's Respite Center
1733 N.E. 162nd St.
North Miami Beach, FL 33162
(305) 940-3510

Hialeah Adult Center
(305) 883-8020

Hospice, Inc.
4770 Biscayne Blvd., Suite 200
Miami, FL 33137
(305) 576-9333

Hospice Care
300 E. Bay Dr.
Largo, FL 34640
(813) 586-4432

Hospice of the Florida Keys
P.O. Box 6558
Key West, FL 33041
(305) 294-8812

Housing & Urban Development Community Services
1401 N.W. 7th St.
Miami, FL 33125
(305) 644-5100

HRS Aging and Adult Services
Judy Powers, Program Administrator
401 N.W. 2nd Ave.
Miami, FL 33128
(305) 377-5021

HRS Background Screening Coordinator
701 S.W. 27th Ave., Suite 712
Miami, FL 33135

HRS District Administrator
401 N.W. 2nd Ave.
Miami, FL 33128
(305) 324-2432

HRS Food Stamps
1605 S.W. 107th
Miami, FL 32165
(305) 227-5060

HRS Human Services Program Specialist
(Medicaid eligibility determinations)
1320 S. Dixie Hwy.
Coral Gables, FL 33146
(305) 663-2094

Jack Orr Senior Center
Jack Orr Plaza (305) 579-5588
Musa Isle Senior Center (305) 638-6684

JESCA Senior Center
2350 N.W. 54th St.
Miami, FL 33142
(305) 638-5500

Jewish Vocational Nutrition Program
420 Lincoln Rd., Suite. 320
Miami Beach, FL 33139
(305) 673-5106

Jewish Community Centers
Dave & Mary Alper
11155 S.W. 112th Ave.
Miami, FL 33176
(305) 271-9000
and
610 Espanola Way
Miami Beach, FL 33139
(305) 673-6060
and
Michael-Ann Russell
18900 N.E. 25th Ave.
North Miami Beach, FL 33180
(305) 932-4200

Kendall Adult Day and Respite Care Center
9820 N. Kendall Dr.
Miami, FL 33176
(305) 271-6311

Legal Services of Greater Miami, Inc.
(305) 576-0080
Culmer/Overtown Neighborhood (305) 573-0354
Miami Beach (305) 672-2004

Little Havana Activities & Nutrition Centers, Inc.
(305) 858-0887

Locktowns Community Mental Health
(305) 653-6594

Long-Term Care Ombudsman Council
Deborah Sokolow, Coordinator
1320 S. Dixie Hwy.
Coral Gables, FL 33146
(305) 663-2085

Lutheran Ministries of Florida Older Workers Program
225 2nd St.
Miami Beach, FL 33139
(305) 674-8111

Meals on Wheels
395 N.W. 1st St., Rm 208
Miami, FL 33128
(305) 347-4650

Medicare Alzheimer's Project (MAP)
151 N.E. 52nd St.
Miami, FL 33137
(305) 754-8665

Memory Disorders Center
University of Miami School of Medicine
Center on Adult Development and Aging
1400 N.W. 10th Ave., Suite. 314-A
Miami, FL 33136
(305) 324-2775

Methodist Senior Center Hot Meals Program
400 Biscayne Blvd.
Miami, FL 33132
(305) 371-3392

Metro Dade County Transit Administration
(Reduced fares for elderly/handicapped)
(305) 375-4644

Miami Beach Jewish Senior Center Outreach
(305) 673-0062

Miami Jewish Home and Hospital for the Aged Care Line
5200 N.E. 2nd Ave.
Miami, FL 33137
(305) 576-5533

Miami Lakes Catholic Hospice
14100 Palmetto Frontage Rd., Suite 370
Miami Lakes, FL 33016
(305) 822-2380

Miami Springs Senior Citizen Center
(305) 887-5442

Monroe County Medical Society
Box 1210
Marathon, FL 33050

Monroe County Social Services
1315 Whitehead St.
Key West, FL 33040
(305) 294-8468

Mount Sinai Medical Center
Automated Response Monitoring System (ARMS)
4300 Alton Rd.
Miami Beach, FL 33140

Community Outreach Programs
(305) 674-2312

ELDERCARE
(305) 674-2052

Geriatric Psychiatry Program
(305) 674-2940

Physician Referral Service
(305) 674-2273

Project Sinai
(305) 674-2437

Senior Care Program
(305) 937-2022

Social Services Department
(305) 674-2750

Transportation services
(305) 674-2155

Wien Center for Alzheimer's Disease and Related Memory Disorders
(305) 674-2543

National Parkinson Foundation Adult Day Care Center
1501 N.W. 9th Ave.
Miami, FL 33136
(305) 547-6666

Neighborhood Family Services
New Horizon Community Center 7505 N.E. 2nd Ave.
Miami, FL 33138
(305) 754-7342

North Dade Adult Day Care
60 N.E. 166th St.
North Miami Beach, FL 33162
(305) 940-0075

North Miami Beach Public Library Support Group
164 St. and 16th Ave.
North Miami Beach, FL 33162
(305) 948-2970

North Miami Foundation Companion Respite Care
(305) 893-1467

North Miami Foundation for Senior Citizens Services, Inc.
(305) 893-1450

Parent Care & Senior Support Services
743 N. Powerline Rd.
Deerfield Beach, FL 33442
(800) 352-7359

Pathways Project/Miami Jewish Home & Hospital for Aged
151 N.E. 52nd St.
Miami, FL 33137
(305) 751-8626

Perrine Senior Program
(305) 233-9134

Project Help (Transportation—North Miami residents only) (305) 948-2902

Project Independence*
151 N.E. 52nd St.
Miami, FL 33137
(305) 751-3095
and

Channeling*
151 N.E. 52nd St.
Miami, FL 33137
(305) 758-0021

* Both Project Independence and Channeling offer evaluation of needs and design of an individualized package of services, including skilled nursing, respite care, meals, speech, physical and occupational therapies, homemaker/personal care, escorts, housekeeping, and physician visits. They are affiliated with the Miami Jewish Home and Hospital for the Aged.

Riviera Presbyterian Church Alzheimer's Support Group
5275 Sunset Dr.
Miami, FL 33143
(305) 666-8586

Senior Citizen Activity Center of Homestead
(305) 245-4934

Senior Community Service Employment Program
American Association of Retired Persons (AARP)
3750 S. Dixie Hwy.
Miami, FL 33133
(305) 447-0020

Senior Ride
(Miami Beach residents only, for medical *appointments*)
(305) 673-8658

South Beach Family Center/YWCA
(305) 305-9922

Southeast Florida Center on Aging
Florida International University
151st St. and Biscayne Blvd.
North Miami, FL 33181
(305) 940-5550

Southwest Social Services
(305) 261-6202

Surfside Community Center
(305) 866-3635

Harold and Patricia Toppel Rehabilitation Center
Miami Jewish Home and Hospital for the Aged
151 N.E. 52nd St.
Miami, FL 33137
(305) 751-8626, Ext. 461

University of Miami Center on Aging Memory Disorder Clinic
(305) 547-4082

Veterans' Administration Adult Day Care
South Shore Hospital
630 Alton Rd.
Miami Beach, FL 33125
(305) 672-2100

Veterans Administration Hospital and Nursing Home Care
1201 N.W. 16th St.
Miami, FL 33125
(305) 324-4455

Veterans' Affairs Service Office
(800) 368-5899

Villa Maria Adult Day Care Center Support Group
1050 N.E. 125th St.
North Miami, FL 33161
(305) 891-9751

Visiting Nurse Association of Dade County
3900 N.W. 79th Ave.
Miami, FL 33166
(305) 477-7676

West Dade Adult Day Care
5895 W. Flagler St.
Miami, FL 33144
(305) 261-5278

West Miami Senior Center
(305) 266-1122

Legislative Offices

Florida House of Representatives, Aging and Human Services Committee
424 House Office Building
Tallahassee, FL 32399-1300
(904) 488-8315
Representative Art Simon, Chairman
Tom Batchelor, Staff Director

Florida Senate, Health and Rehabilitative Services Committee
400 Senate Office Building
Tallahassee, FL 32399
(904) 487-5340
Sen. John McKay, Chairman
Bev Whiddon, Staff Director

U.S. Senate, Special Committee on Aging
G-41 Dirksen Bldg.
Washington, D.C. 20510-6400
(202) 224-5364
Sen. David Pryor, Chairman
Theresa M. Forster, Staff Director

National and State Organizations

Administration on Aging
Fernando Gil-Torres, Secretary
U.S. Department of Health and Human Services
330 Independence Ave. S.W.
Washington, D.C. 20201
(202) 619-0724

Alzheimer's Disease and Related Disorders Association
919 N. Michigan Ave., # 1000
Chicago, IL 60611
(312) 853-3060, (800) 621-0379

Alzheimer's Florida Information Line
(800) 330-1910

American Association of Homes for the Aging
901 E St. N.W., Suite 500
Washington, D.C. 20004-2037
(202) 783-2242
Sheldon L. Goldberg, President

American Association of Retired Persons (AARP)
601 E St. N.W.
Washington, D.C. 20049
(202) 434-2277
Horace B. Deets, Executive Director

AARP Legal Council for the Elderly
601 E St. N.W., Bldg. A, 4th Floor
Washington, D.C. 20049
(202) 872-4700

American Bar Association Commission on Legal Problems of the Elderly
1800 M St., N.W.
Washington, D.C. 20036
(202) 331-2297
Nancy Coleman, Staff Director

American College of Health Care Administrators
325 S. Patrick St.
Alexandria, VA 22314
(703) 549-5822
Richard L. Thorpe, Executive Vice President

American Foundation for the Blind
15 W. 16th St.
New York, NY 10001
(212) 620-2000
Carla Augusto, Executive Director

American Geriatric Society, Inc.
770 Lexington Ave., #300
New York, NY 10021
(212) 308-1414
Linda Hiddemen, Executive Vice President

American Health Care Association
1201 L St. N.W.
Washington, D.C. 20005
(202) 842-4444

American Society for Geriatric Dentistry
1121 W. Michigan St.
Indianapolis, IN 46202
(317) 264-8845

American Society on Aging
833 Market St., #512
San Francisco, CA 94103
(415) 882-2910

American Speech-Language-Hearing Association
10801 Rockville Pike
Rockville, MD 20852
(301) 897-5700
Dr. Frederick T. Spahr, Executive Director

Asociacion Nacional Por Personas Mayores
3325 Wilshire Blvd., #800
Los Angeles, CA 90010
(213) 487-1922

Association for Gerontology in Higher Education
1001 Connecticut Ave., Suite 410
Washington, D.C. 20036
(202) 429-9277

Better Hearing Institute
(703) 642-0580, (800) 424-8576

Cancer Care and the National Cancer Care Foundation
1180 Ave. of the Americas
New York, NY 10036
(212) 302-2400
Harvey I. Newman, Executive Director

Catholic Golden Age
430 Penn Ave.
Scranton, PA 18503
(717) 342-3294

Children of Aging Parents
2761 Trenton Rd.
Levittown, PA 19056
(215) 945-6900
Louise G. Fradkin and Micra Liberti, Directors

Commission on Legal Problems of the Elderly
American Bar Association
1800 M St. N.W.
Washington, D.C. 20036
(202) 331-2297

Department of Veterans Affairs
810 Vermont Ave., N.W.
Washington, D.C. 20420
(202) 233-4000, (800) 282-8821

Displaced Homemakers Network
1625 K St., Suite 300
Washington, D.C. 20005
(202) 467-6346

Elder Abuse
State of Florida (to report suspected cases of abuse)
(800) 962-2873

Elder Craftsmen
135 E. 65th St.
New York, NY 10021
(212) 861-5260
Barbara B. Stires, Executive Director

Elderly Referral Panel/Florida Bar Lawyer Referral Service
(904) 222-5286

Equal Employment Opportunity Commission
2401 E St., N.W.
Washington, D.C. 20507
(202) 634-6922, (800) 872-3362, TDD (202) 634-7057

Florida Bar Center
600 Apalachee Pkwy.
Tallahassee, FL 32301-8226
(800) 342-8011

Florida Alzheimer's Disease Initiative
Department of Elder Affairs
1317 Winewood Blvd.
Bldg. 1, Rm. 317
Tallahassee, FL 32399-0700
(904) 922-2078, ext. 117

Florida Council on Aging
P.O. Box 1046
Tallahassee, FL 32302
(904) 222-8877

Florida Department of Elder Affairs
(904) 922-5297

Gerontological Society of America
1275 K St., N.W., Suite 350
Washington, D.C. 20005-4006
(202) 842-1275

Health Care Financing Administration
(800) 638-6833

International Association of Gerontology
Duke University Medical Center
Box 2948
Durham, NC 27710
(919) 684-3416

Legal Assistance
Florida Center for Governmental Responsibility
University of Florida
Holland Law Center
Gainesville, FL 32611
(904) 392-2237

Legal Services for the Elderly
130 W. 42nd Street, 17th Floor
New York, NY 10036-7803
(212) 391-0120
Jonathan A. Weiss, Director

National Association for Home Care
519 C St. N.E.
Washington, D.C. 20002
(202) 547-7424

National Association of the Deaf
814 Thayer Ave.
Silver Springs, MD 20910
(301) 587-1788

National Association for Hearing and Speech Action
10801 Rockville Pike
Rockville, MD 20852
(301) 897-5700
Russell Malone, Executive Director

National Association of Independent Living Centers
2111 Wilson Blvd., #405
Arlington, VA 22201
(703) 525-3406

National Association of Professional Geriatric Care Managers (NAPGCM)
655 Alvernon Way, Ste. 108
Tucson, AZ 85711
(602) 881-8008

National Association of Retired Federal Employees
1533 New Hampshire Ave. N.W.
Washington, D.C. 20036-1279
(202) 234-0832
H.T. Charles Carter, President

National Association of Senior Living Industries
184 Duke of Glouchester
Annapolis, MD 21401
(301) 263-0991

National Association of State Units on Aging
1225 I Street
Washington, D.C. 20005
(202) 898-2578

National Caucus and Center on Black Aged
1424 K St. N.W., #500
Washington, D.C. 20005
(202) 637-8400
Samuel Simons, President

National Citizens' Coalition for Nursing Home Reform
1224 M Street N.W., Suite #301
Washington, D.C. 20005
(202) 393-2018

National Council on Teacher Retirement
P.O. Box 1882
Austin, TX 78767-1882
(512) 335-0055

National Council on The Aging, Inc.
409 3rd Street S.W.
Washington, D.C. 20024
(202) 479-1200
Dr. Daniel Thursz, President

National Eye Care Project
P.O. Box 6988
San Francisco, CA 92401-6988
(800) 222-3937

National Hispanic Council on Aging
2713 Ontario Rd. N.W.
Washington, D.C. 20009
(202) 265-1288

National Indian Council on Aging, Inc.
P.O. Box 2088
Albuquerque, NM 87103
(505) 242-9505
Curtis D. Cook, Executive Director

National Institute on Aging
National Institutes of Health
Bldg. 31, 9000 Rockville Pike
Bethesda, MD 20892
(301) 496-1752

National Institute of Mental Health
5600 Fishers Lane
Rockville, MD 20857
(301) 443-4513

National Senior Citizen Law Center
1816 H Street N.W., Suite #700
Washington, D.C. 20006
(202) 887-5280

Parkinson's Education Program
3900 Birch St., #105
Newport Beach, CA 92660
(714) 640-0218

Senior Community Service Employment Program
Division of Older Worker Programs
U.S. Department of Labor
200 Constitution Ave. N.W., Rm.N-4641
Washington, D.C. 20210
(202) 219-5904

Social Security Administration
6401 Security Blvd.
Baltimore, MD 21235
(800) 772-1213

Veterans Administration
Florida Regional Office
P.O. Box 1437
144 First Ave. S
St. Petersburg, FL 33731

Villers Foundation
1334 G St. N.W., Suite 3
Washington, D.C. 20005
(202) 628-3030

Geriatric Research

Florida Institute of Technology
Claude Pepper Institute for Aging and Therapeutic Research
150 W. University Blvd.
Melbourne, FL 32901
(407) 768-8000, ext. 7329

Florida International University
Southeast Florida Center on Aging
North Miami Campus
North Miami, FL 33181
(305) 940-5550

Florida State University
Institute on Aging
Tallahassee, FL 32306-4053
(904) 644-2831

University of Florida
Center for Gerontological Studies
3355 Turlington Hall
Gainesville, FL 32611
(904) 392-2116

University of Miami
Center for Adult Development and Aging
1425 N.W. 10th Ave., Suite 200
Miami, FL 33136
(305) 548-4593

Center for the Study of Aging and Human Development
Duke Geriatric Evaluation and Treatment Clinic
Box 3469, Duke University Medical Center
Durham, NC 27710
(919) 684-3176

State Units on Aging

Alabama
Commission on Aging
R.S.A. Plaza
770 Washington Ave., Suite #470
Montgomery, AL 36130
(205) 242-5743

Alaska
State Agency on Aging
Older Alaskans Commission
P.O. Box 110209
Juneau, AK 99811
(907) 465-3250

Arizona
Aging and Adult Administration
P.O. Box 6123
1789 W. Jefferson
Department 950-A
Phoenix, AZ 85007
(602) 542-4446

Arkansas
State Office on Aging
Donaghey Bldg., Suite 1412
7th and Main St.
Little Rock, AR 72202
(501) 682-2441

California
Department on Aging
Health and Welfare Agency
1600 K St.
Sacramento, CA 95814
(916) 322-5290

Directory

Colorado
Aging and Adult Services Division
Department of Social Services
1575 Sherman St., 10th Floor
Denver, CO 80203
(303) 866-3851

Connecticut
Department on Aging
175 Main St.
Hartford, CT 06106
(203) 566-7725

Delaware
Division on Aging
Department of Health & Social Services
1901 N. Dupont Hwy.
New Castle, DE 19720
(302) 577-4660

District of Columbia
District of Columbia Office on Aging
1424 K St. N.W., 2nd Floor
Washington, D.C. 20005
(202) 724-5622

Florida
Deprtment of Elder Affairs
1317 Winewood Blvd.
Tallahassee, FL 32301
(904) 922-5297
E. Bentley Lipscomb, Secretary

Georgia
Office of Aging
Department of Human Resources
878 Peachtree St. N.E., Rm. 632
Atlanta, GA 30309
(404) 894-5333

Hawaii
Executive Office on Aging
Office of the Governor
State of Hawaii
335 Merchant St., Rm. 241
Honolulu, HI 96813
(808) 586-0100

Idaho
Office on Aging
Statehouse, Rm. 108
Boise, ID 83720
(208) 334-3833

Illinois
Department on Aging
421 E. Capitol Ave.
Springfield, IL 62706
(217) 785-2870

Indiana
Department on Aging and Community Services
402 W. Washington
Indianapolis, IN 46207
(317) 232-7020

Iowa
Commission on Aging
914 Grand Ave.
Jewett Bldg.
Des Moines, IA 50319
(515) 281-5187

Kansas
Department on Aging
Docking State Office Building, 122-S
915 S.W. Harrison
Topeka, KS 66612-1500
(913) 296-4986

Kentucky
Division for Aging Services
Bureau of Social Services
275 E. Main St.
Frankfort, KY 40621
(502) 564-6930

Louisiana
Office of Elderly Affairs
P.O. Box 80374
Capitol Station
Baton Rouge, LA 70898
(504) 925-1700

Maine
Bureau of Maine's Elderly
Department of Human Services
State House, Station 11
Augusta, ME 04333
(207) 624-5335

Maryland
Office on Aging
State Office Building
301 W. Preston St., Rm. 10004
Baltimore, MD 21201
(410) 225-1100

Massachusetts
Department of Elder Affairs
1 Ashburton Pl.
State Office Building
Boston, MA 02108
(617) 727-7751

Michigan
Office of Services to the Aging
611 W. Ottawa, N. Tower 3rd Fl.
P.O. Box 30026
Lansing, MI 48909
(517) 373-8230

Minnesota
Board on Aging
444 Lafayette Road
St. Paul, MN 55155-3843
(612) 296-2770

Mississippi
Council on Aging
455 N. Lamar Street
Jackson, MS 39206
(601) 359 6770

Missouri
Office of Aging
Department of Social Services
P.O. Box 1337
615 Howerton Court
Jefferson City, MO 65102
(314) 751-3082

Montana
Department of Family Services
P.O. Box 8005
Helena, MT 59604
(406) 444-5900

Nebraska
Department on Aging
P.O. Box 95044
301 Centennial Mall S.
Lincoln, NE 68509
(402) 471-2306

Nevada
Division of Aging Services
Department of Human Resources
1665 Hot Springs Rd., #158
KinKead Bldg.
Carson City, NV 89710
(702) 687-4210

New Hampshire
Division of Elderly and Adult Services
115 Pleasant St.
Annex Building 1
Concord, NH 03301
(603) 271-4680

New Jersey
Department of Community Affairs
CN 807
S. Broad and Front St.
Trenton, NJ 08625
(609) 292-4833

New Mexico
State Agency on Aging
LaVilla Rivera Bldg.
224 E. Palace Ave.
Santa Fe, NM 87501
(505) 827-7640

New York
Office for the Aging
Agency Bldg. 2
Empire State Plaza
Albany, NY 12223
(518) 474-4425

North Carolina
Division on Aging
Department of Human Resources
693 Palmer Drive, CB # 2931
Raleigh, NC 27626-0531
(919) 733-3983

North Dakota
State Agency on Aging
Department of Human Services
1929 N. Washington
Bismarck, ND 58501
(701) 224-2577

Ohio
Commission on Aging
50 W. Broad St.
Columbus, OH 43266
(614) 466-5500

Oklahoma
Special Unit on Aging
Department of Human Services
P.O. Box 25352
Oklahoma City, OK 73125
(405) 521-2281

Oregon
Senior Services Division
Human Resources Department
500 Summer St. N.E.
Salem, OR 97310-1015
(503) 378-4728

Pennsylvania
Department of Aging
400 Market St.
Harrisburg, PA 17101
(717) 783-1550

Rhode Island
Department of Elderly Affairs
79 Washington St.
Providence, RI 02903
(401) 277-2858

South Carolina
Commission on Aging
400 Arbor Lake Dr., Suite B-500
Columbia, SC 29223
(803) 735-0210

South Dakota
Office of Adult Services and Aging
Division of Human Development
Richard F. Kneip Bldg.
700 N. Governor's Dr.
Pierre, SD 57501-2291
(605) 773-3656

Tennessee
Commission on Aging
706 Church St., Suite 201
Nashville, TN 37243-0860
(615) 741-2056

Texas
Department of Aging
P.O. Box 12786
Capitol Station
Austin, TX 78711
(512) 444-2727

Utah
Division of Aging Services
120 N. 200 W., Box 45500
Salt Lake City, UT 84145

Vermont
Office on the Aging
103 Main St.
Waterbury, VT 05671-2301
(802) 241-2400

Virginia
Office on Aging
10th Floor
700 E. Franklin St.
Richmond, VA 23219

Washington
Bureau of Aging and Adult Services
Department of Social and Health Services, OB-44-A
Olympia, WA 98504
(206) 753-2502

West Virginia
Commission on Aging
State Capitol
Charleston, WV 25305
(304) 558-3317

Wisconsin
Department of Health and Social Services
1 W. Wilson St.
Madison, WI 53702
(608) 266-2536

Wyoming
Commission on Aging
 Bldg., Rm. 139
Cheyenne, WY 82002
(307) 777-7986

About the Contributors

Judith A.S. Altholz, Ph.D., is currently in private practice as a psychotherapist, trainer, and consultant in Tallahassee. Prior to entering her practice, Dr. Altholz was on the faculty of Florida State University School of Social Work for 14 years and previous to that was on the faculty of Duke University Medical Center.

Marian Bruin, A.C.S.W., B.C.D., is a professional geriatric care manager and the president of Star Systems Consultation and Training, Inc., in Tampa. She is nationally recognized for her work in advocacy, care management, and long-term care planning.

Pamela Cody is a nursing home marketing director and admissions coordinator in Palm Harbor. She is the founder and former president of the Alzheimer's Disease and Related Disorders Association, Tallahassee chapter. She has completed course work in psychology at Florida State University.

Marie Cowart, R.N., Ph.D., is director of the Florida State University Institute on Aging. Cowart holds a doctorate in health care administration from Columbia University, and a master's from Tulane University.

Margaret Lynn Duggar, M.S., Ed., served as a member of the Florida Pepper Commission on Aging. From 1984–1989 she served as assistant secretary of aging and adult services for the State of Florida, where she was responsible for planning and overseeing programs and services for older Floridians. Duggar also served as executive director of the Area Agency on Aging for North Florida and of the Senior Society Planning Council, and was chair of the Elderly Access to Health Care Task Force, 1988-89. She holds bachelor's and master's degrees from Florida State University.

C. Colburn Hardy is a graduate of Yale College and, after taking early retirement as a public relations executive with an international corporation, started a second career as a writer. He has authored 27 books on investments, money management, and retirement. In Florida, he has been an active volunteer on aging committees including the Florida Commission on Aging. He lives in West Palm Beach.

Gema G. Hernandez, Ph.D., is an associate professor at the Nova University School of Business and Entrepreneurship and a consultant to the Little Havana Activities and Nutritional Centers, the Miami Jewish Home and Hospital, the Channeling Project, the University of Miami Center on Aging and Developmental Disabilities, and Partners in Wellness, Inc. An ethno-gerontologist, Hernandez provides training to area agencies on aging nationwide on the importance of recognizing clients' cultural values and beliefs in their programs. Her contribution to the *Florida Caregivers Handbook* includes several caregiver profiles.

Tann Hunt, J.D., is a Tallahassee attorney. She has published a book and several articles on family law matters. Hunt is a graduate of the Florida State University College of Law. Prior to beginning her career in law, she taught English at Florida State University.

Robert J. Kassan, M.D., had a private medical practice in rheumatology in White Plains, New York, for more than 35 years. His medical degree is from the George Washington University School of Medicine. He currently serves as the medical director of a South Florida "medivan" project, which provides health care services to the poor elderly.

Jayne LaRue, M.S.W., is a recent graduate of the Florida State University School of Social Work. She has worked with aging clients in home and institutional settings as a certified nursing assistant and as a private care manager. She recently accepted a social work position with the Veterans Administration in St. Petersburg.

Sarah S. Morrill, M.S.W., is the former director of Apalachee Community Mental Health Services in Tallahassee. Since her retirement in 1986, she has remained active in the community, as a consultant and volunteer, currently serving on the Department of Elder Affairs Advisory Committee. Her contribution to the *Florida Caregivers Handbook* includes a number of the caregiver interviews and profiles.

Creston Nelson-Morrill is a journalist and author specializing in the economic and social aspects of health care delivery and related insurance issues. She is the president and publisher of HealthTrac, Inc., a health policy research and publishing company in Tallahassee. A graduate of Florida State University, Nelson-Morrill also has completed graduate course work in law and health economics.

Thomas W. Poulton is the former editor of the *HealthTrac Tallahassee Report on Health Care Issues*. He also oversaw a multi-user computer network for a Florida hospital association and served as a consultant on legislative and administrative issues related to health care. Poulton holds a bachelor's degree from the University of Florida and is completing a law degree at the University of Florida.

Karen Ring, M.S.W., L.C.S.W., is a licensed clinical social worker in private practice in Tallahassee, where she has served as a field instructor at Florida State University and as a consultant to Big Bend Hospice. She has more than 10 years' experience in mental health and social work. Ring holds bachelor's and master's degrees from Florida State University.

George F. Slade, M.D., serves on the faculty of the Florida A&M University School of Allied Health Professionals and is a former faculty member of the University of Florida School of Medicine, Department of Neurology. Slade also serves as a consultant to the Division of Children's Medical Services of the State of Florida. He earned his degree in medicine from Emory University.

Dawn T. Pollock holds a master's degree in organizational communication and marketing from Florida State University. She has more than 10 years experience in program development and administration and is the founder of Concept Associates, Inc., a consulting firm specializing in the management of services and nonprofit firms. She also served as the director of a demonstration project to help defer nursing home placement by providing health care services to elderly persons and their caregivers.

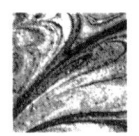

About HealthTrac Research Group, Inc.

HealthTrac Research Group, Inc., (HRG) was incorporated in 1991 to conduct public policy research in the health care field; to establish pilot projects and programs benefiting the elderly and their caregivers; and to disseminate related information to the public in the form of articles, brochures, books, and audio and video tapes. Issues related to caregiving and long-term care are two of the areas identified by the board of directors as the focus of early initiatives.

The *Florida Caregivers Handbook, Revised Second Edition*, will serve as the foundation for our efforts to provide education and support to caregivers. Fund-raising efforts are on-going to ensure broad distribution of the Handbook and to support development of educational videos and other related programs. HRG is a 501(c)(3) charitable, tax exempt organization and all contributions are tax deductible.

For additional information on HRG, please write us at P.O. Box 13599, Tallahassee, Florida, 32317.

NOTES

NOTES

ORDER FORM

FOR ADDITIONAL COPIES OF FLORIDA CAREGIVERS HANDBOOK

Single copy price: $14.95

shipping/handling: $3.00

Florida residents please add 7% sales tax: $1.05

Total: Florida residents $19; non-residents $17.95

Name _____

Address _____

City / State / Zip _____

Order from:

Healthtrac
BOOKS
P.O. Box 13599
Tallahassee, FL 32317